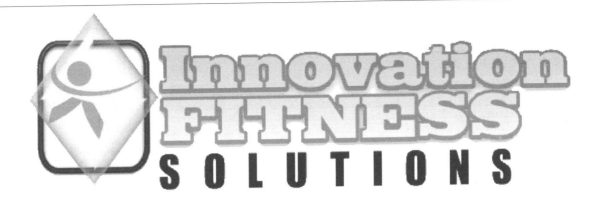

90 days to a new you

The Mental and Physical keys to long term success.

Transform your thinking.
Transform your body.
Transform your life.

By: Robert J. DeVito

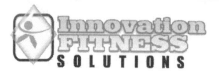

Foreword:

It is estimated that America is 4,000,000,000 Lbs. overweight. We now consume 300 calories more per day than just 25 years ago. For the first time in generations our children are estimated to have a shorter life span than we have. Health Care for heart disease, diabetes and other weight related issues is in the billions of dollars per year and people are generally unsatisfied with the quality of their lives. This book can be a staple part of your solution to a newly transformed and invigorated being.

I have been a friend and colleague of Robert DeVito for 15 years. His passion and dedication is unparalleled in his quest to transform individuals. This passion is a gift he inherited from within to give to you.
By utilizing the principles and strategies of this book, you will undoubtedly begin on a path of personal transformation.

Jason Morgan
President – Dynamic Health and Fitness
www.dhfstudio.com
www.dhfonline.net

Dedication:

To all of the thousands of clients and Fitness Professionals that I have had the honor of working with over the past 15 years, I thank you. The lessons in this book come from you.

To my wife Misty Mae, you are my reason. Your strength and courage are an inspiration to me.
To my son Anthony, you are my world and I am so proud to be your Da Da.
I love you both with all my heart.

-Robert

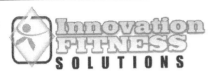

Table of Contents

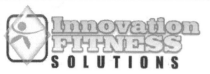

**2016 Hours. 90 days. 12 weeks. 3 Months. This is a lot of time to make BIG changes.
90 days to a NEW YOU!**

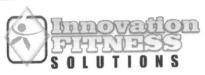

Introduction

I have been fortunate enough in my life to work one on one with thousands of individuals; all of which had the same goal; to transform their body and self-esteem. I have come to the conclusion that in order to do so it takes a *Transformation in your Thinking*.

It is estimated that America is 4,000,000,000 Lbs. overweight. Americans consume 300 calories more daily than just 25 years ago and we move less do to technological increases… There is a substantial amount of information available to you on all of the health concerns and potential diseases, ailments and loss of self esteem that are associated with being overweight or obese. In this book we will tackle the issues from a *Solution Based* standpoint, not from a Problem Based view.

Belief is the basis in all action. Transform your beliefs and you can change your behaviors. If you change your behaviors you can attain the results you are after.
Attain your results and you transform your life.

What is dramatic, transformational change?

Usually people do things in half measures or an All or None mindset. Take a look back now at all of the little changes that you have made in the past to get you where you are now. Are you comfortable with each of these changes now? Yes, probably you are. But while they happened you may have had doubts. Once all of these changes are instituted you are looking at a whole new you, a new outlook, a new body, a new way of looking at eating as well as exercise. A new outlook on life and on what you can achieve.

Some change can be harder...but very important

Most change in life that is really serious and permanent comes from radical changes in beliefs, thoughts and actions. When you make a break from the past and change the way that you look at all things in your life you are changing a paradigm and you never need look back. I have been in points in my life in the past where I would look at some kind of exercise, lifestyle change, relational change or long held belief and would kind of chuckle saying "No, I couldn't do that" or "No. I won't do that." and six months later I am at that point.

The other thing that I see is that most great people are normal people and that we can push ourselves to succeed. The only thing that it takes is to really make a difference in your outlook, attitude and what you think that your limits are. Once you remove your limiting beliefs you can fill your life with possibilities and the education needed to make change last.

This book is all about one simple philosophy: Transformation.

Focus on today and tomorrow

What you do today shapes your tomorrows. Focus on today and tomorrow. Try and look at the limitations that you have put in your way. I always fall back on how my bad knee stops me from running, but instead I walk every day.

Do you have any "bad knees" that are holding you back?

Do you smoke and want to quit?

Do you have a weight problem and have tried every diet but none of them have worked?

Do you get down on yourself when you don't do things perfectly?

Be Solution Based, not Problem Based. It is easy to give up. It takes strength, commitment and dedication to persevere. Start to think about your possibilities - not your limitations.

We must learn to recreate our thought process and recreate our habits in order to *Transform Our Body* and *Transform our Life* long term. In reality, every diet ever created works for a short time. Diets have one thing in common; they manipulate you into eating fewer calories daily. Sadly, the methods utilized by most of these diets are not intended for long term results. They capitalize on your motivation and temporary dislike with yourself. In the following pages we will evaluate what it will take for you to create a plan that is specific to your success. The book represents a process, a system to success. We do not prescribe nor recommend a certain diet or exercise plan. Rather, we suggest altering your thinking to alter your habits. Ultimately, your habits (how you live your life) determine who you are. We will progressively move from one point to another. We suggest preparing yourself by taking things slowly. You will not lose your weight all at once and you most likely will not be successful with tackling every change that needs to be made all together. If you have attempted similar methods with similar thinking then we strongly urge you to reconsider the belief that short term methods can and will lead you to long term results.

We will take into account the physical, mental and emotional needs to be successful in a long term program. We have often seen rapid results achieved by drastic methods. These repeated attempts and short lived results usually see the dieter rebound hard. Either gaining most or all of their lost weight back and in many instances gaining more than they lost, even though they were "Dieting"! Over the next 90 days you will have a detailed plan that takes into account all aspects of success. Physical change is easy to attain but very difficult to maintain if the foundational education is not present.

The text that follows holds the keys to be successful. You will lose fat and weight, you will increase "tone" and you will look and feel better. Along the way you will have setbacks; your weight loss will slow down and potentially even stall completely for a while AND you will have great successes! We promise that if you follow our suggestions and you commit to doing the work the rewards will be there.

Always think about how your choices effect what you do today and in the future.

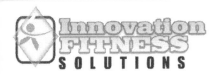

Your Strategy for Success

Weight management is a simple five word strategy: Eat Less and Move More. The key to long term fat loss is to create an energy deficit while giving yourself as much health as you can stand. The *IFS* philosophy for weight management is **R.P.M. A → B (Realistic, Progressive and Maintainable)** and incorporates three easy to remember bullets:

> 1) Make "Better Bad Food Choices"
> 2) Surprise Exercise
> 3) Minimize Damage

There are **R**ealistic, **P**rogressive and **M**aintainable strategies that fit into your lifestyle. Once we master the chosen strategies we can move forward with those and add more. This will continually produce results over time.

Your changes and habits must fit your goal

I often hear from new clients and multiple people a day that they "Eat Healthy" and I do not doubt it. Many health and weight conscious people tend to eat healthier than those that are not. There is a clear misunderstanding in regards to food and weight loss. I tend to think about it this way:

Weight Gain and loss is controlled by your quantity of food (How Much) and Health is controlled by your Quality (How Good). There are plenty of individuals that "Eat Healthy" but cannot budge their weight. Ask yourself two simple questions:

1) Do you know how many (Quantity) calories you consume daily?
2) Do you know how many (Quantity) calories you burn daily?

If you cannot successfully answer these questions you are relying on guesswork. Remember:

Weight control is about **Quantity**

Health Improvement is about **Quality**

If your primary goal is Weight Loss I suggest controlling your calorie intake and expenditure while eating as healthily as you can stand. Over time as you lose weight and have success you will naturally gravitate toward making healthier food choices and new exercise habits. Focus on your goal.

Goals and Expectations:

Properly managing your expectations with realistic short and long term goal setting is one of the important keys to your success. Many times we set goals for ourselves that are too aggressive. Although we are very aggressive from the start, the road we choose is usually too difficult to maintain. This generally leads to the viscous cycle of start and stops dieting and exercise fads. Setting short term goals is especially important because long terms goals do not allow us to celebrate achievement along the way, thus leaving us feeling discouraged. This book is based on the long term principle "because you can do it and keep doing it, makes it the right plan for you".

You cannot lose 50 lbs. without losing 1 lb first.

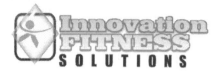

Through the principles and strategies in this book you will come to realize that getting to your goals is not as difficult (or as easy) as popular marketing tells you. There is no magic, but it does take planning and consistency. It is not necessary to be so restrictive and hard on yourself both physically and mentally. The reality is that life gets in the way. In order for us to get to the bottom of what works, we must realize that everything works! But what is optimal for one person is different for everyone else. Just as we all have different careers, values, preferences, etc... we all will have different eating and exercise plans.

There are a few things that you can be sure of:
1) There is no "magical fattening or fat burning foods".
   All food can help you gain or lose weight.
2) The same goes for "miracle exercises". They do not exist.
   There is not one exercise or workout that you can do to achieve permanent results.

EVERYTHING works and then it stops working. The workout that allowed us to lose 10 Lbs., the bottle of pills that temporarily shed a few more, the restrictive diet that ended up being way too hard to follow; all of these methods are a short-term fix to a long-term goal.

The first lesson is: **CONSISTENCY**. Consistency can be achieved by following *Realistic, Progressive and Maintainable* strategies for long-term results. This is the cornerstone of the *IFS* weight loss philosophy.

In the long run you are free to choose what you do or do not do. The decisions you make and the habits that you form determine your outcome. That means that you are in control, you are responsible for your actions. This is both a powerful and an empowering statement.
The lesson is: *You* **CONTROL** *your environment; your environment does not have control over you.*

Finally, the third lesson is: **PLAN.** You have to be aware of your surroundings and make a plan that is realistic for you. Any good plan has a direct route and an infinite number of alternate routes. We all know that perfection does not exist, so stop trying to hold you to the perfect plan. You ultimately will fail. For long term success, I recommend that you think in terms of "better bad" not perfect. Look for ways to enjoy life's little pleasures but be accountable for your actions. Look for ways to move more during the day, not only in the gym but at the office and at home as well. Most importantly, stay positive. Remember that one meal does not "blow it" and missing one workout does not destroy your week or make it impossible to achieve the goal that you chose. The only way you will not succeed long term is by giving up.

Do not use short term methods for long term goals.

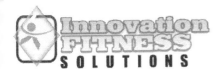

Realistic Progressive and Maintainable Strategies for Success

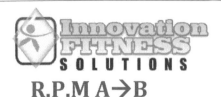

R.P.M A→B

**Realistic, Progressive and Maintainable Strategies
Philosophy Defined:**

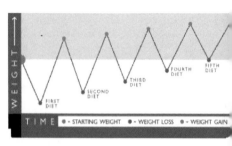

Setting the stage for success

Dieting and/or exercising to lose weight can be difficult mentally
and physically. If you review the chart above and you identify
with its' flow you also know that repeated, failed attempts leave
you drained emotionally and feeling hopeless. You may give the next fad diet or magical exercise
plan a chance, maybe even believing that it may work for you. Generally though, frustration mounts
after another failed method. Most of this frustration is due to the ineffective and inaccurate quick
results that have been promised to you. Losing weight and gaining it back causes true long term
weight/fat loss to become more difficult. Anytime you have lost significant weight (10 lbs/ +) you
have lost some muscle tissue. Muscle tissue loss causes your metabolic rate (your ability to burn
calories) to go down. This results in you having to eat less food to maintain your weight or makes
weight gain even easier.

Your plan: For Now or Forever?

Your habits determine your outcomes. This is why determining what you can do forever, not just for
now is important. Can you eliminate or drastically reduce foods that you like from your diet? Will
you really not drink any alcohol ever again? Can you exercise daily for hours for the rest of your life?
Will you always rely on prepackaged foods in cardboard boxes? We have had experience with
thousands of individuals, many of which that had or wanted to attempt these "cures" for their
unwanted weight gain.   Some of these people got very lucky and succeeded with their chosen method
but most (98%) are not successful at keeping their weight off for more than one month or two…

Is it Motivation or Commitment?

Why is it that it is so easy to buy the newest diet book or subscribe to the thinking in the magazines
that usually contradict themselves month to month? Do you remember a few years ago when you were
told to not go near carbohydrates because they were the reason that you were gaining weight? But now
we're told carbohydrates are OK as long as they're the "right" ones…

Do you recall back in the 1990's we were told to eat all of the carbohydrates we wanted to as long as
we avoided Fat at all costs? We have been told that we can lose all of our weight very quickly if we
just don't eat after 8:00PM, we have been told to make sure we combine our meals a certain way and
to never eat other foods together. We have been told to eliminate entire food groups, specific foods, to
only eat miracle foods and to exercise as soon as we wake up in the morning or just by exercising our
stomachs for 7 minutes a day we'll miraculously look how we want… I believe the reason we fall prey
to these "cures" is timing. We become disgusted with ourselves and very, very motivated to change
our appearance. A solid understanding of neither all the reasons for weight gain nor the best strategies
for weight loss have been available we had to rely on half truths and false promises.

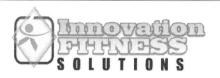

Now, as the numbers of obese and overweight/underactive individuals continue to increase and the related diseases do too, research has offered multiple breakthroughs in improving health and fitness levels. If we combine that with what is known about the process of change a solution begins to emerge.

Commitment is everything in this process. This process can be fun and it can be much less taxing on you than your previous attempts. An understanding that you will have setbacks and you will have tough days and you will eat foods that you feel that you shouldn't have and that workouts will be missed is essential to your long term success. Preparing for overcoming obstacles and avoiding plateaus will keep you on track.

Eat Healthy and Exercise Regularly
Gaining weight and low self-esteem go hand-in-hand. When we eat too much we feel bad about ourselves. These negative emotions are often **a** root cause of eating problems. To gain a healthy weight it is essential that you escape this cycle. *Create New Habits to become a NEW YOU.*

Healthy weight loss requires that you do two simple things - eat healthily (within your limits) and exercise regularly. Up to now you may have tried to lose weight by embarking on restrictive diets and this is probably why you still need to lose weight. Restrictive diets set you up to fail. It is not a matter of IF, but when you will stop that method.

You may lose weight in the short-term on a restrictive diet but you will probably find yourself putting it back on before too long. Too often you will find yourself back at square one, or worse. Failure will only add to any lack of self-esteem you may have.

Whether one increases or decreases the size of their fat stores day to day depends upon the relationship of calories consumed and absorbed versus energy expended on metabolism and daily activity. If you were in a caloric deficit at the end of the day, then more fat would have come out for energy than went in for storage, so your fat stores would be decreased. However, if you were in caloric excess, then more would have gone in than went out, so your fat stores would increase. As you can see, having an understanding of calorie balance will be important to your success. Your body needs material to work with to cause fat stores to increase and stay that way. That material is the calories we eat.

> **Keep in mind that there are really only two ways to change something:**
>   1) Stop or start doing something(s) completely
>   2) Do more or less of something(s) that already exists

Create New Habits

Some methods that have been shown to not succeed for most people:
Low Fat Foods Do Not Work
You cannot lose weight using Low Fat Diets. Low fat foods have been popular for more than 15 years, but yet our society is getting more overweight as each year passes. This fact alone should tell you that eating a purely low fat menu is not the answer to losing weight.

Low Calorie Diets Do Not Work
You won't lose weight using a Low Calorie Dieting Plan either. In fact, eating low calories is the worst thing that you can do to your body, since that will only slow down your body's metabolism and make reaching your goal more difficult (low calorie diets may allow a few pounds of weight loss for the first few days, but then after that fat loss comes to a halt --- known as a dieting plateau). You will not achieve the toned, athletic look you desire by starving yourself.

Low Carbohydrate Diets Do Not Work.
You'll probably find it extremely difficult to get lean using a Low Carbohydrate Plan. Versions of these diets have been popular for more than a decade now, but the problem with this method is that they are too strict and TOO HARD TO FOLLOW for any length of time. Low carb menus tend to rob your body of too much energy (carbohydrates) and make it nearly impossible to remain consistent long enough to have lasting effects. This is why so many dieters find it difficult to follow a strict low carbohydrate menu.

The Solution: What does work?

R. P. M. A --> B
The keys to long term weight loss success are Control, Consistency and Prior Planning!
Use Long term planning for Long term success! Focus on short and long term goals utilizing Realistic, Progressive and Maintainable (R.P.M.) strategies. This method should allow you to have control over food selections and pace of progress. You will see and feel results quickly and maintain these results through our educational system.
Get educated: Take Control.

Change Bank Theory: Everything is cumulative
Have you ever saved your change? You begin with an empty container and slowly add your pocket change to it until it's full. At first you don't have much at all, a few quarters, a handful of pennies and a couple of nickels and dimes… But, over time, a few weeks or months the change begins to accumulate and add up. This is the philosophy to take with you. We are creating ways to increase our calorie expenditure within our health club workouts to maximize the time spent and we are finding ways to burn a few pennies, nickels and dimes (low calories burning activity) in our daily lives.
We are looking for ways to shave a handful of calories by reducing our food intake here… making a different choice there…

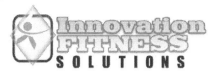

A small change repeated over time will yield huge results.

Realistic: simply means that the change must fit your current lifestyle. If it does not you will not keep doing it and return to your previous habits. Choose foods that you enjoy eating and will continue to eat. Choose a fitness plan that you can and will stick to. The "Perfect Plan" is not very good if you will not do it.

Progressive: Choose the habits to change that you know you can change. When you "own" those then you can add more. There is no need to tackle everything at once. Do what you can do, not what you can't. A → B then B → C.

Maintainable: The success comes from the continuation of habits. Choose against short term methods for long term goals. Strategies that you can do daily and repeatedly will always win out over "quick fixes".

Keys to success:
1. Know how much food and how many calories you are eating.
2. Change your "Gym" workouts frequently to prevent your body from adapting and slowing calorie burn.
3. Nourish your body with nutritious foods and a Multi-Vitamin.
4. Energy is a choice! Find reasons to move when you would not normally.
5. A calorie expended cancels a calorie consumed.
6. Rome was not built in a day. Have an Action Plan.
7. Be kind to yourself.
8. Stay Positive!

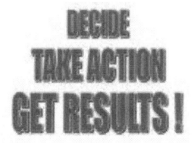

Transform Your Thinking.
Transform Your Body.
Transform Your Life.

13
www.InnovationFitnessSolutions.com

How to use this book:

I suggest re-reading the introduction on a weekly basis. Repetition will create a true understanding of the methods and material and function as an aid to get you back on track when things get off track…which they will from time to time.

In the rear of this book are daily fitness tips. Keep this book handy and read the tips every day. Highlight the tips that really strike you and refer to them often. Another suggestion is to read the *Quick Reference* Guide Daily. There is a ton of Daily Questions to keep you on track and helpful reminders to keep you on track.

During the first month I recommend that you read all of the support material (Chapter: Support Material) and perform the exercises in the 'Days 1-30 Workbook'. The information contained in the support material acts as an owners' manual for your body.

Be sure to log on to www.InnovationFitnessSolutions.com
Click the Tab titled **<90 Days to a New You>** and enter the code **(90NEWYOU).**
You will find printable forms of:

- Daily Food Log
- Weekly Exercise Planner
- Grocery Shopping list
  - Cardiorespitory and Resistance Training Workouts with Photos
- Weekly Report Card
- Daily Fitness Tips
- Motivational Quotes

The **first 30 days** of this book are all about setting the stage for success. We will implement simple and immediate strategies to get you burning more calories and eating less. Knowing how you arrived at where you are and the initial steps to take to reverse the trend are essential. Weeks 1 and 2 should be spent on choosing the simplest habits to change for good. Weeks 3 and 4 are to be spent altering more habits. This time period is where a substantial amount of progress gets made very, very quickly. Motivation will most likely remain very high during this time.

The **second 30 days** are geared toward standardizing and planning your movement program in your health club and taking advantage of whatever time you have outside during "real life". Whereas a few simple "tricks" work well during the first phase of weight loss, time allows the body to adapt and more adjustments must be made. We'll find ways to burn more calories and new tips and "tricks" to take less in without feeling deprived.
Your weight loss will begin to stabilize at this point. You will still be losing weight, just not as quickly. This is natural and to be expected. DO NOT try to force the issue by "Dieting" or exercising like a maniac! Keep the **R.P.M.** Principles in mind. This is a Progressive plan. Not an All or Nothing plan.

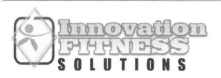

The **last 30 days** are all about maintaining the progress that you have had and continuing the trend. It will just be slower... The body is fighting for you to return to your "former self" at this point. It is a matter of survival for your body. It is not concerned about your appearance and is desperately trying to figure out how to get you to eat more. You may notice your cravings a little higher and more intense but we have added steps to prevent that from derailing your success. At this point we'll discuss in depth what your body is doing to you and how to stop it in its' tracks. Whereas motivation is probably high early on because weight loss is easy and seems to be falling off of you, progress slows and becomes more difficult with time. You have to commit at this point.

I suggest reading and rereading each chapter of this book at the beginning of each 30 day period. The lessons will be reinforced and you will learn more and implement more strategies from each read through.

Read the book in its' entirety (up t your current month) at the beginning of the month. Reread the monthly plan and lessons each during the month and spend 10-15 minutes daily reading the current months plan and lessons. Repetition breeds success.

-Robert J DeVito

"The way to get started is to quit talking and begin doing."
-Walt Disney

We all have two choices:
To accept who and where we are in life
Or
To strive for what we can become and where that can take us!
-Mark Stevens

"Nothing is particularly hard if you divide it up into small jobs."
– Henry Ford

"Our thoughts create our behaviors."
-R. DeVito

15

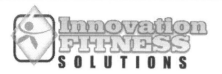

Days 1-30
Getting Started:
<u>The Mindset</u> and <u>The Tools</u>

Transform Your Thinking.
Transform Your Body.
Transform Your Life.

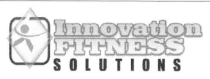

Days 1-30

Getting Started: The Mindset and The Tools

It is important to start off in the right direction (and at the correct speed) and have a full understanding that long term success is not about finding the magical diet or exercise plan. You will not find the perfect workout plan and your friend who quickly lost 15 pounds did not discover the magical solution even if they are losing weight rapidly right now (watch them next week and next month).

Start where it starts. You have to have a commitment to changing the habits that got you where you are. Discover them and consistently and systematically change them. There is enough reliable information available about how people change for good and the entire process of long term change to know that there is no magical solution. We'll deliver some simple strategies to aid you in the fight against fads and mental madness. Let's discuss some of the things that we have discovered working with more than 10,000 clients. We have seen the good, the bad and the plain insane.

Vision, Belief, Persistence, Learning
The first essential to success is having a vision. Do you know what exactly you are trying to achieve? The more specific that your goals are the more real your vision becomes. Try taking a few moments to write down who you want to be. Try not to stick only to physical goals but include athletic performance and family activity goals. In my experience I have seen more clients be successful when there is a goal that is "bigger than just vanity". Having goals (in addition to the weight loss), such as spending more quality time with your children playing, or running a 5K are essential. There are numerous studies that have shown when people write their goals down they are more likely to achieve them (40% more). It doesn't take much time and it only helps. Furthermore, make a portable cheat sheet to carry with you. Once you have determined who you want to be then carry that person with you. It's a helpful reminder of what you are accomplishing.

Second: Believe that you can do this.
The chances are pretty good that you have lost a decent amount of weight before. Maybe you have kept it off and wish to lose more or, like many of us your losses were only temporary and you've regained most if not all of your lost weight. That was the past. There were different circumstances and a different understanding of what it takes to be successful. Believing in yourself in the face of past failures shows that you are strong. Staying positive where most others are negative will help you remain focused.
We have found that simply believing that you will be successful will have a tremendous impact on your actual success. You will rebound from setbacks quicker and stay positive more often.

> **Believe you can**

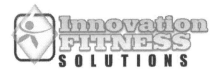
Third: Persistence:

One of my favorite sayings is "Don't let perfect get in the way of good". There are numerous environmental and lifestyle landmines that you'll face. Your kids will want Mc D's and you'll eat a few fries, Valentine's Day, Halloween and Easter bring chocolate by the wheelbarrow, summer brings cotton candy and hot dogs etc… Striving for perfection simply sets you up for difficult, tedious times that mentally torment you. Striving for perfection will only lead you to frustrations and failure. You will eat foods that you feel like you shouldn't. You'll drink alcohol and miss workouts. It will not prevent you from being successful. Persistence means you will accept these 'mistakes' and move on from them.

Understanding that we are humans and we are not perfect allows you to enjoy life's little pleasures and still succeed. Control yourself and indulge occasionally, but be smart and do not over-indulge. That's just gluttonous and counter-productive, it won't help you.

Realistic Goal Setting and Properly Managing your Expectations are two more keys to Long-Term Success. Remember, "Don't let perfect get in the way of good".

> Life is not a diet.
> Life is life.

> **"Don't let perfect get in the way of good."**
> **Striving for perfection will only lead you to frustrations and failure.**

Last: Learning

You need to keep a journal. Journaling your Food and Fitness allows you to do your detective work. It will reveal trends (Good and Bad) and allow you the ability to change the habits that are hurting your progress. When you do not have documented information you are reliant on memory and guesswork. Can you recall everything that you've eaten and drank for the last 2 weeks? I can't either, but it is incredibly important information if you want success. Your habits will determine your outcomes and knowing your calorie intake along with your trends will aid you to make logical decisions. Journaling will help you determine your best practices list.
A list of things that you do that work for you is a key tool to long-term success. Keep an honest journal.

VISION:	Who do I want to be? Attributes and Attitudes	What are your most beneficial habits?
		1.
1.		2.
2.		3.
3.		4.
4.		**What do you feel you should change first?**
5.		1.
6.		2.
7.		

You cannot reach a goal if you do not know what it is.

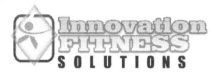

Catch Yourself Succeeding

Immediate and Easy Changes: Do these now for Instant Success.

Now that we have our heads on straight, we're thinking logically and we are committed to this process let's get all of the tools we need for success. Many of us fill with the fear of the idea of facing ourselves in the mirror on a daily basis. If this is the case, then now is the time to embark upon a complete fitness overhaul. A few well-placed strategies can pay off much greater than a major approach to shedding some of the winter insulation. Change your way of thinking to win long term. **Control, consistency and planning** will guide you along the way.

1) Breakfast.
Eat it every day. Breakfast boosts your metabolism and prevents mid morning ravenous hunger. Avoid hunger at all costs! I have never seen anyone make a solid, logical food decision while they were starving. Beginning with breakfast and insuring that you eat at least 3 meals and 1-2 snacks everyday will aid you in avoiding these mindless choices that we regret later. What will you eat for breakfast tomorrow? How about the next day? After that?

2) Complimentary sessions:
If you are a member of a Fitness Center go see a Weight Management Specialist to find out how many calories you can eat daily and how many you need to burn. Use your Complimentary Personal Training Sessions to revamp and reenergize your workouts. Find new strategies to burn more calories and challenge your stability, balance, coordination and strength. Get into the mindset of "controlled chaos" workouts. Use everything in the Fitness Center and at home to keep moving. Remember: Change = Change
Even if your Trainer is a Novice they will still be able to teach you a few new tricks.

3) Food Journal, Nutrition Scale
Visit www.InnovationFitnessSolutions.com and purchase a food Journal and a Nutrition Scale. When you eat foods (and liquids) with labels it is easy to accurately determine how many calories you are consuming, but what about foods without labels? Did you REALLY eat 3 oz. of chicken or was it actually 4.5 oz.?
If you skip a regular 20 ounce soda and save 250 calories, switch from whole milk to skim milk and save 50 calories a cup; go for regular coffee instead of a blended drink and save 300 calories. Remember, small changes (R.P.M. A → B) tend to be the most effective method over time. Having the ability to do your calorie detective work will be essential as you move through your transformation.

Plan your Day

19

4) Celebrate your achievements

"We have 50-60,000 thoughts a day. 90% of them are negative."   -Deepak Chopra

Carry your 'cheat sheet' and begin to write down your list of successes.
Write down the fact that you had an extra workout this week; ink the note that you only had 2 drinks this week instead of 4-5. All positive steps should be rewarded. Weight loss is a long hard road. There are tons of outside obstacles and many times "life gets in the way". If you keep moving forward and incrementally changing habits from bad to better you will start to see positive changes for good.

> **Focus on progress, not perfection.**

5) Supplement your diet.
Let's face it, no one eats properly everyday and exercise actually increases your nutrient needs. Take a Multi Vitamin for nutritional insurance and to help stave off muscle tissue loss.
Use the non stimulant based Fat Loss Aid during workouts to maximize calorie expenditure during your cardio workouts. The ingredients help you to use fat as fuel during exercise.
If you want to maximize your results then this is the way to go.

6) Don't try to tackle everything at once
Pick two or three things that you can change this week that will have a great impact on your results. This is usually enough to jump-start your program and begin to see results. Remember that Rome wasn't built in a day and you will not see dramatic changes overnight. Use photos to judge your progress along with how your clothes are fitting and circumference measurements. Don't rely too much on the scale readings, they tend to move up and down a little everyday, so only check your weight once every two weeks or even better yet only once a month. This will give you a clear understanding of what's happening.

7) Get Active
Find ways to include "Surprise Exercise". We have included a chart for non gym based activities from standing instead of sitting through athletic activities. Take advantage of the weather and get outside and do a few activities that you enjoy. The more you move the more calories you burn. This will allow you to lose weight faster or eat more food.

8) Make Up Your Mind.
Decide you are going to change and accept it. Partial commitment will lead to partial results. Just because you ate well and exercised for a week, do not expect to be at your goal weight. As the weeks go by, your progress will pick up momentum and changes will become much more visible. Consistency is the key. Have you ever read the story of *The Tortoise and the Hare*? I would love for you to use this example in your weight loss quest. Slow and steady wins the race! Set realistic goals. As a rule of thumb my suggestion is to expect a 1 pound weight/fat loss per week.

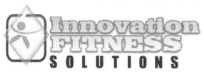

9) Honestly Assess What You Are Considering Eating.

Ask yourself, "Will eating this food get me closer or further from my goal?" If the answer is further, then make a better choice. Everyone loves French fries or donuts, but eating these things on a regular basis will make it very difficult to attain your desired shape. Creating more "food decisions" and making yourself accountable is another one of the keys to consistency. Think before you eat.

10) Eating for Pleasure is Normal.

Our ability to make rational food choices have been destroyed by the manufacturing of foods that serve no purpose other than to taste unbelievably good. Maybe the burgers and fries, pizza, 600 calorie coffee drinks and chips were ok when we were younger, but as we age, most of us do not get enough daily movement to be able to eat for taste alone.

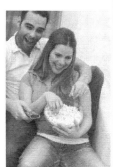

11) Food Choices Are a Habit.

Replace poor food choices with "Better Bad Food Choices". This act in and of itself will help reduce our calorie intake. As we progress we can continue to make better and healthier choices. The longer we do it the better our new habit will be. You will find that you will feel better when you eat properly and you will ultimately discover that the bad food makes you feel badly. Seriously, try this! Most of us do not actually know what it feels like to feel good – only bad and less bad. After a few weeks of truly feeling good your habits will naturally change forever.

12) Do Not Buy Junk Food.

Similar to the previous recommendation, this includes the elimination of poor food choices from your home. If you do not have it in the house, you cannot eat it. A potential disaster can be avoided. This also increases the number of food decisions you will have to make. If you need to go out and get it, you probably will not eat it as often. When you finally eat these foods as treats, as they were originally were intended, that is what they will become.

> **If you do buy junk food here is 3 ways to increase the # of food decisions!**
>
> 1. Buy snack sized bags (100 calorie)
> 2. Tape the bag after eating and put it in the back of the cabinet.
> 3. Put a Post-It note on or near the food: "Do I REALLY want this?"

13) Eat Consistently Throughout the Day.

Drastic calorie reduction and long periods without food will lead to a decline in your metabolic rate, resulting in low energy. Ultimately, you will eat again and the choices you make will not be controlled. Skipping meals leads to the creation of hunger and hunger makes people do stupid things.

Your ability to make wise food choices becomes difficult when hunger kicks in.

Smaller, more frequent meals and snacks (four to six times a day) will help stave off hunger by keeping blood sugar levels under control. Be honest with yourself. If you work with a trainer, be honest with them as well. A half of a cookie still contains calories. If you take little bites of different foods throughout the day, it adds up. Fruit juice has calories. Sugar and milk in coffee or tea has

---

Change your habits and you'll change your life!

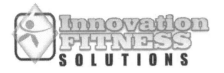

calories. Alcohol has calories. Eating while standing still counts, it all counts. Count it. If you don't we will still know. An "Honesty covenant" is the best policy.

14) **Include Resistance Training.**
Even if your goal is fat loss, this aspect of your training is extremely important. Resistance exercise burns calories, strengthens bones, reduces risk of heart disease, improves strength and coordination for daily activities, makes you look better and makes fat loss easier. Once thought of as just a "get big" form of activity, is now well researched to benefit all fitness goals.

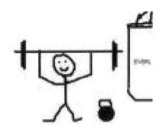

> SURPRISE Exercise!
> Move for the sake of moving.

15) **You Have to Move.** Incorporate more movement into your daily activities, even if you already spend an hour, maybe two, exercising. At best, this is 1/12 of the day. If you can find a way to work more movement into the rest of your waking hours, just think how much of an impact that can have. Go for a walk at lunch or during a break. Try parking farther away than you do now. Take the stairs. Stand up for 5 minutes every time you answer the phone. Walk down the hall at work rather than use the intercom. Use the speakerphone at work and pace around the room as you talk.

16) *Mix It Up!* Most of us have certain machines or exercises that we really enjoy because we are really good at it. Unfortunately, when you get good at something, your body adapts. When your body adapts, you tend to burn less calories doing that activity. So, every two weeks or so, change up your cardio and exercise routines.
Training the same way trains you to stay the same.

17) *Cravings.* When you're faced with cravings for sweets or other favorite foods satisfy your craving with a small portion of the food you desire. Eat it slowly, savor every bite, and then resist the urge to reach for more. Another option: Chew on a piece of sugarless gum. Studies have shown that this can be a calorie-free way to satisfy your urge for something sweet.

18) **Drink plenty of water** or other calorie-free beverages. People sometimes confuse thirst with hunger. So you can end up eating extra calories when an ice-cold glass of water is really what you need. Add in citrus or a splash of juice, or brew infused teas like mango or peach, which have lots of flavor but no calories. South Beach and Crystal Light make no calorie flavor additions as well.

> **Eating every 3-4 hours will keep your energy stable.**
> **NEVER go 5+ hours without eating something.**

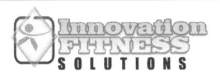

19) ***Fill Boredom with anything but food!*** Food can become a time filler when you are bored. Try to motivate yourself and get active during periods of boredom. This will benefit your weight loss efforts twofold: 1 – You'll take in fewer calories. 2 – You will burn more calories.

20) **Grocery Shopping** is best done while you are not hungry. Be sure to use a list and focus on the foods that you know will help you get to your goal. Avoid the snack aisle if you need to. Purchase all of your "staple" foods first and then go back for your "goodies". I bet you will find the need for them to be less if you wait until the end of your shopping trip. Purchase plenty of vegetables and fruits.

21) **Be prepared for roadblocks, speed bumps, plateaus, and bumps in the road**. Adopt the mindset of resiliency. You know that not everything will go smoothly and you know that you will be able to bounce back from any setback. Planning for these instances will save you countless frustrations. Be mentally strong and committed to the process of weight loss. It is not a quick process.

22) **Know the difference between water loss and fat loss.** As discussed in the section on 'Body Weight Range' you will have fluctuations in your weight from day to day. It is important to not get "too happy or excited" when the scale reads a few pounds down and not get "too upset" when the scale is on the high side. Add a bit of logic to this emotional roller coaster. There are 3500 calories in each pound of fat. If you lost 3 lbs yesterday, did you figure out how to burn 10,500 extra calories? The same concept applies in the opposite direction. Did you eat 10,500 EXTRA calories yesterday? This fluctuation is normal. Treat it that way.

23) **Maximize your metabolism to maximize your results.** Commit this 'mantra' to your memory and act on it daily. Wake up, eat breakfast, move for 10-15 minutes, walk around your office all day, stand when you can instead of sitting, eat frequently, and eat deliberately and wisely.

24) **Commit to cook meals at home at least twice a week.** Quite literally I am one of the worst cooks in this world. I have dozens of people that have taken me up on the offer to let me cook for them once, and only once. But, I still continue to cook. I get to control the ingredients and the portions, I get to minimize the outside temptations and I get to feel good about creating the menu and the meal. It is a win-win. You can also cook extra and freeze your meals into small, single serve containers for times when you don't feel like cooking or even eating out.

25) **Meal replacement options.** If you have ever choked down a 'Protein Bar' in the past in an effort to stay the course you know that these are convenient options to maximize meal frequency and control over eating. You also know that many of them taste like the bottom of your trash can. There is good news! Engineered food technology has come a long way in the past few years and you can actually find somewhat 'healthy' and decent tasting Meal Replacement Bars, cookies and muffins. I would suggest choosing the Food Bars as opposed to the Meal Replacement Shakes for Fat/Weight Loss. Shakes do not require as much digestion as the Bars/Cookies. Choose those to maximize your metabolism.

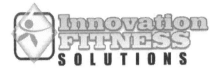

Borrowed from Brian Tracy:
The 100 Absolutely Unbreakable Laws of Business Success

The Law of Direction:
Successful people have a clear sense of purpose and direction in every area of their lives.
The steps to success:
1) *Decide exactly what you want.*
2) *Write it down* in clear, specific, detailed language.
3) *Set a deadline.* If the goal is large set sub-deadlines.
4) *Make a list* of everything that you can think of to do to achieve your goal.
5) *Organize your list into a plan* based on priorities and sequence.
6) *Take action!* Do not delay.
7) *Do something every day (*no matter how small) that moves you toward the goal.

Catch Yourself Succeeding

Studies have also shown that we tend to unknowingly eat more calories in the following situations:
• Food is presented in large quantities (restaurants, parties)
• A wide variety of food is present (buffets, all you can eat)
• More people are present
• Being distracted and doing something else (watching TV)
• Eating out of large packages (bag of chips, tub of ice cream)
• Tempting foods are within reach and within eyesight

You can find a number of healthier options that have less calories, fat and sugar but still leave you satisfied. Some ideas:
• Replace regular chips with baked chips or soy chips.
• Replace ice cream with frozen yogurt or sorbet
• Replace full-fat cookies with fig newtons
• Replace soda with flavored sparkling water

Starting Measurements:
Your first step is to record the following measurements: weight, resting heart rate, body fat and circumference measurements. Write down your numbers and be sure to write down the date. You'll use this same chart every four weeks or so to record new numbers to track your progress.
You may also wish to get starting strength measurements as an additional way to gauge your success.

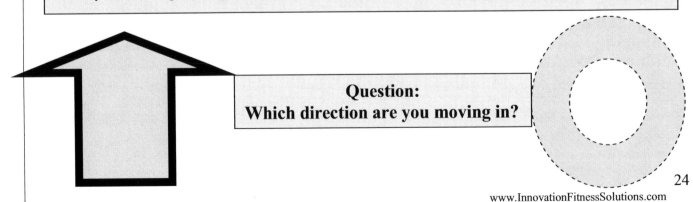

Question:
Which direction are you moving in?

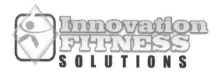

5 MORE WAYS TO SHAVE CALORIES WITHOUT COUNTING THEM

The average restaurant dinner is around 2000 calories...this could be a problem! Here are some ways to make sure that you do not over do it while eating out.

1. *Decrease Your Speed of Eating.* It takes 15-20 minutes for your stomach to stretch and send a signal to your brain that says you are full. If you eat too fast you will eat too much and that leads to "eating to pain". At this point you know you overdid it. In addition, do not "pre-load" your fork. Wait until you are done chewing and swallowing the first bite before you load your fork for the second.

2. *Pick Your Favorite – "Cheat Well".* Do not just eat it because it is there and it is a holiday. Only eat what you really love. If sweet potatoes are your thing then have some, but pass on the mashed.

3. *"One bad apple does not ruin the bunch" or "The Egg Theory".* If you buy a dozen eggs and one breaks on the way home you don't throw the whole dozen in the garbage. Every meal is its own egg and if you break one egg do not throw out the dozen. <u>Eating is cumulative</u> and nothing you do today will make you wake up at 400 pounds. When you break an egg, just go to the next meal and eat what you should and add more movement to cancel those calories!

4. *"Calorically Cheapen" Your Meal.* There are no "good" or "bad" foods, only "Healthy" and "Unhealthy". In the context of money, high calorie foods are "expensive" and low calorie foods are "cheap". When you are making your mashed potatoes use skim milk instead of half and half...you just *"calorically cheapened"* that dish. If you are going to eat a piece of pie...forego the ala mode and you just *"calorically cheapened"* that dessert. This will only help <u>minimize damage</u> and help keep you on track because you are still adding in your favorite foods.

5. *"Pre Eat" before you go out to dinner.* Eat a regular breakfast and lunch then eat something right before you go to dinner. Now the "battery on your will-power" will be fully charged. If you go into the meal too hungry you will eat faster and longer. So, prevent yourself from getting too hungry. Stay consistent to stay on track.

Stock your kitchen with healthy convenience foods.

Having ready-to-eat snacks and meals-in-minutes staples on hand sets you up for success.
You'll be less likely to hit the drive-through or call in a pizza order if you can make a healthy meal in 5 or 10 minutes.

- 94% fat-free microwave popcorn (20-25 calories per cup, and you can make it in two minutes or less)
- Frozen vegetables and Bags of pre-washed greens, Frozen Healthy Meals.
- Canned diced tomatoes and/or beans
- Whole-grain wraps or pitas
- Pre-cooked grilled chicken breasts and a few containers of pre-cooked brown rice
  Within minutes, you can toss together a healthy medley.

To prevent unconsciously over eating, follow these tips:

- Eat and only eat. Avoid being distracted during mealtimes or snack times.
- Eat from smaller plates, bowls and glasses.
- Portion out your food and avoid "family style" eating or eating out of the package.
- When you dine out, control the portion sizes by sharing meals or packaging some to take home right away.
- During social occasions, decide on what you're going to eat and stick to it. Otherwise you'll graze mindlessly.
- Limit your alcohol intake. Alcohol tends to stimulate appetite and reduce your awareness of what you're eating and how much.
- Keep snacks, treats and tempting foods out of reach.

Surprise Exercise of the week:

Avoid all escalators, elevators and moving walkways all week.
Take the stairs whenever possible.

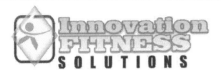

Here are the Steps to Making a Big Change

1. Believe It is Possible

Your success is determined more by your belief than by any other factor. Regardless of how hard you plan and work at it, if you do not believe you can succeed, you will not. Conversely, regardless of the obstacles facing you, if you believe you can succeed, you will.

2. Commit to Change

Where does the power to make the change and overcome barriers come from? The power is yours as soon as you make a commitment. A deep conviction, or willingness to do whatever it takes to succeed, releases the power to act and crush all barriers in the way.

3. Act As If You Are Already The person You Want To Be

Immediately after making a commitment to change, act as if you are already the person you want to be. For in the days and weeks that follow, your new behavior will crystallize into a new habit. Moreover, your new behavior will cause others to treat you as the person you want to be. And their new way of looking at you will reinforce your belief that you have changed.

4. Celebrate Your Success

Congratulations on your success! Now it's time to celebrate. When you do so, it helps seal your new identity. But when you celebrate, do so in a manner that adds to rather than takes from your life. Treating yourself to dinner with friends is an example of adding to life, but celebrating by getting drunk with friends only invites trouble and the possibility that you may begin to unravel the good you have already done.

Copy these steps
and hang them
on your
refrigerator!

Believe, Commit, Act, Celebrate

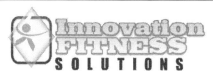
Days 1 – 30: Articles
Different Goals have different needs

Fat Loss, *Health and Fitness*, and *Sports and Performance* goals all place different demands on the body. They range from the amount of sleep required to the number of meals and calories eaten daily to what they are made of (Protein, Carbohydrates and Fats) and how many meals you eat per day. It is slightly different for everybody. If you add in your genetic predisposition for where and how much fat you hold, your given metabolism, food preferences and dislikes plus your attraction or aversion to exercise it can be exhausting and de-motivating to try and figure all of these items out for yourself.

My advice: DO NOT GIVE UP! That is one surefire method to fall short of your fitness goals.

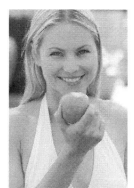

FAT LOSS
Fat matters, carbohydrates count but calories are the bottom line! Do not buy into the myth that some foods are fattening and others are not. It is not true. Every food can help make you gain weight and every food can help you keep it off. The amount of ingested has to be less than the total calories burned or you will get bigger eating sunflower seeds and grapefruits. It just does not matter!

HEALTH AND FITNESS
The more consistent and the healthier the choices that you make the better you will feel. I suggest 30-45 minutes of cardiovascular work 3-4 times weekly + 2-3 strength training sessions weekly. In addition, maintaining a diet of consistently balanced foods along with your exercise routine will help you achieve your goal with ease. Your body will thank you for it and your mind will as well. When we choose healthy options we give our body the fuel it needs to keep going strong throughout the day, fight off cellular damage and be mentally sharp.

SPORTS AND PERFORMANCE
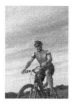
Eat often, eat well and eat balanced! The timing of your pre and post workout meals is crucial to your success. Eating 45-60 minutes pre-workout is essential to providing the energy necessary for optimum performance. A post workout meal consisting of a 4:1 ration of carbohydrate to protein is important for recovery. In addition, optimal rest (6-8 hours of sleep) and the proper training intensity are essential too. Try not to work out more than 3 days consecutively if your intensity level is above a 7.5 on a scale of 1-10.

RESULT
In my opinion one of the strongest variables someone can change is to get out of daily result and into process. It is a BIG PICTURE way of looking at your goals and your goal setting. Everything matters but mistakes will be made and they will be corrected. Nothing is impossible and a great plan makes for great successes.

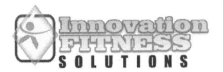

Having a Positive Attitude Will Help You with Losing Weight

How you feel about your efforts to lose weight is very important. If you have a positive attitude about your goals and the plan to reach them then you will increase your chances of success.

Too many people make the mistake of doing all or nothing when it comes to weight loss. One day they don't exercise at all and eat most things in sight. The next day they are going to work-out a lot and only eat healthy foods.

A consistent and flexible plan of action will trump an "All or Nothing" effort over time.

For example, if you have committed to exercising every day for the past two weeks and eating healthily, treat yourself by going to a movie you have been dying to see. Or perhaps treat yourself to a new outfit when you lose 10 pounds or enjoy a day at the spa. You deserve to be rewarded for all of your efforts.

Your goals will be more achievable if you break them down. Remember to give them a time frame as well.

Use affirmations:

Everyone remembers the great Saturday Night Live skit: Daily Affirmations with Stuart Smalley. "I'm good enough, I'm smart enough and gosh darnnit, people like me!"

It worked for him and it can work for you too. Begin with two or three saying that you can repeat to yourself to remind you of why you're doing this (Reason), your specific daily, weekly or monthly goals (Goal) and your plan for success for the day (Plan).

Find Reasons to Smile.

Affirmations:
Reason, Goal, Plan
1.
2.
3.
4.
5.

Remember:
You control your environment; your environment does not *control* you! Ultimately, you *control* how much you eat or do not eat and how much you move or do not move.

You *control* your outcome!

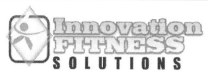

It's Time to learn about our body!

Muscle vs. Fat

All weight loss is not considered equal. This is a mantra to live by as you continue on your weight management program. Though we all are conditioned to determine our success solely by the weight loss shown by the scale, it is much more important to judge our achievements based on our changes in body composition. Besides, do you want to lose weight or lose weight AND change your shape?

Body Tissues

The human body consists of a variety of different types of tissues, lean tissue and fat tissue. The lean tissues include bone, muscle and organs. Muscle and organs are considered metabolically active, whereas fat is metabolically much less active. This means that muscle and organs help to increase your metabolism and burn fat and calories, while fat tissue does almost nothing. Therefore, it is essential to maintain muscle tissue while losing fat, thus the additional movement will increase your metabolism.

Weight

It is important to realize that a pound of muscle is denser and more compact than a pound of fat. It is helpful to think of a pound of fat as a pound of feathers, and a pound of muscle as a pound of iron. The pound of feathers would clearly take up a lot more space than that same pound of iron. By gaining lean body mass (water, bone and muscle) while losing body fat, you will look and feel lighter, your clothes will fit better and your overall sense of well being will improve. In summary, body weight is only one of the many determining factors of success.

Changing your Body Composition

To decrease your percent of body fat, you need to create the right balance between the calories you consume and the calories you expend. The most effective way to do this is to decrease your consumption of calories and increase your activity level.

GENERAL BODY FAT PERCENTAGE CATEGORIES*

CLASSIFICATION	FEMALE % OF BODY FAT	MALE % OF BODY FAT
Essential Fat	10-12%	2-4%
Athletes	14-20%	6-13%
Fitness	21-24%	14-17%
Acceptable	25-31%	18-25%
Obese / Undesirable	32% +	25% +

American Council Exercise

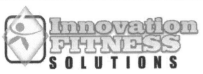

90 Days to A New You

Your Personal Health and Fitness Inventory Worksheet

SMART Goal:	
Specific Can you articulate more clearly what you are trying to do? Can you summarize this in one thought? Refine that thought. Can you summarize a bottom line?	
Measurable How will you know that you attained your goal? Can you quantify or put numbers too your outcome? What affect will your goal have on your life/effectiveness?	
Attainable Is this goal dependent on someone else? Can you rephrase the goal so it only depends on you and not others? Are there any things that would prevent you from accomplishing your goal?	
Relevant What would you like to do? Of the items you mentioned, what things would you like to change most?	
Time-specific When will you reach this goal? Can you give a time limit? How long would it take to create a sustainable habit in this area?	

Daily Surprise Exercise Challenge:

Set an alarm to go off every hour. Take at least 2 minutes to stand up and stretch or walk around.
Begin from the moment you start your day and continue for at least four (or more) hours.

www.InnovationFitnessSolutions.com

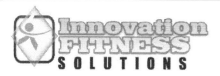

SMART Goal: Your Answers	
Specific	
Measurable	
Attainable	
Relevant	
Time-specific	

Smart Goals Create Intelligent Results

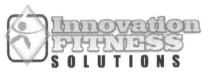

The Innovation Fitness Solution - M.A.P. - My Action Plan:
Vision – Goal – Plan – Execute – Measure – Success!

We have determined our reasons for changing and set our vision. We know we need to be persistent (especially when things are not going "right" and we have full *Faith and Belief* in ourselves that we will be successful. It's a great start! Now, let's look at the HOW's.

Goal –
- ❖ Goals are a simple but funny thing. If they are too grandiose you risk failure, if they are too easy to attain you risk a loss of motivation. Choosing goals (short and long term) takes a realistic evaluation of what you can accomplish and keep accomplishing repeatedly. No one I've met has stated to me that they would like to achieve something and then return to their former selves. | Guesswork will only work Short Term. |

- ❖ Utilize a 4 step Goal Setting approach:
  - o Long Term – Intermediate – Short Term – Immediate
    6 Months   Monthly   Weekly   Daily
  - o Behavioral Modification (Habit Driven)

- ❖ Now do some simple math and project out.
  Look at the long term results of your consistent work.
  If you lose 2 lbs per week for the first 2 weeks   4
  And then 1 lb per week for 4 weeks   +4
  And finally ½ lb per week for 6 weeks   +3 =11
  Staging your results is a much more realistic, maintainable and concise way to manage expectations and stay on target.

Weekly weight loss goal	Daily calories to reduce or burn through activity
½ lb	250
1 lb	500
1.5	750
2	1000

Your Weight Loss Chart:

Week	Weight Loss	Week	Weight Loss
1		7	
2		8	
3		9	
4		10	
5		11	
6		12	

32

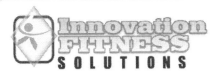

Plan –

❖ You must plan ahead to control your outcome. There is no need to be a fanatic but you will need to know where you can get healthier, lower calorie meals. Over time these new actions will become habits and part of your day. This is where success happens. When you consistently make smarter choices the calorie reductions from food add up and the calorie expenditures from added movement add up too!

❖ *Exercise: Functional Fast Food*

   o Determine your favorite Fast Food Restaurants or Sit Down Establishments and create your "Go To" meals. Hint: Do not choose something you cannot eat repeatedly.

Name 3 places you can get "Better Bad" meals.
1.
2.
3.

Name 3 ways to burn more calories "Surprise Exercise" today?
1.
2.
3.

Execute and Measure–

❖ **Do it!** Are you doing things that bring you closer to your goal daily or just continually thinking about it? Execution is action.

❖ List your habits (Good and Bad). Continue the habits that are helping you and discontinue the habits that are hurting you, but not all at once.

❖ What can you live with? Realistic, Progressive and Maintainable strategies are the key to your success.

❖ Focus on the things that you WILL change not on things that you feel you SHOULD. This will set you up for much better success and give you a positive state of mind.

Know Your "Go To" Meals and Where to Get Them

Transform Your Thinking.
Transform Your Body.
Transform Your Life.

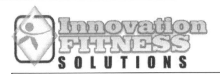

The Mindset to make it work

**To truly achieve health and fitness you must know why you want it.
Take time <u>today</u> to write down 10 reasons why health and fitness is important to you.
Review your list every day.**

<u>**Answer these questions to set your path and put your goals into action!**</u>
1) **What do I want?**
   Make positive statements in terms of what you hope to achieve.
2) **How will I know when I get there?**
   What does my success look and feel like? Create more than just a scale #.
3) **What will I do today, tomorrow, next week, next month to cause my goal(s) to happen?**
   Self initiated and self controlled actions. What R.P.M. changes can be done now? Next week?
4) **Why do you feel prepared to start now?**
   Why do you believe in yourself? Why are you worth this?
5) **What could hold me back or keep me stuck?**
   What has prevented your success in the past? Will you let it again?
6) **How is my energy level? What will I do to improve it?**
   Stretch upon waking, Eat Breakfast, Talk to my partner for 5 minutes to lift my spirit etc…
7) **What would accomplishing these goals do for me?**
   a. Physical Health **b.** Emotional Health
8) **Do I have everything I need (physical, mental, emotional) to achieve my goal?**
   Do you have all the resources necessary to be successful?
   Call me to discuss your plan: (201)951-8080
9) **Do I need to eat differently? How?**
10) **Do I need to act differently? How?**
11) **Do I need to move differently? How?**
12) **What else would change? What would stay the same?**
13) **How will this affect other areas of my life?**
14) **What is my outcome?**
15) **Will these changes truly make me happy?**

Now take this a step further and apply these questions to each Life Quadrant.

Place a Priority # in each Quadrant.

Have fun!

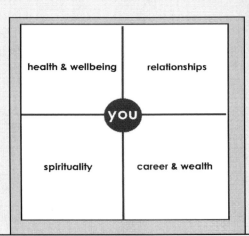

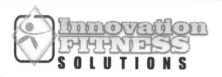

Your 10 reasons:

1.   6.

2.   7.

3.   8.

4.   9.

5.   10.

Answer these questions to set your path and put your goals into action!

1.
2.
3.
4.
5.
6.
7.
8.
9.
10.
11.
12.
13.
14.
15.

Now describe 2-3 Action Steps you can take to affect each Life Quadrant:

	Relationships	Spirit	Wealth
1.			
2.			
3.			

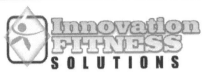
How do you Gain or Lose Weight?

The Law of Thermodynamics

Formal Definitions

- **The First Law of Thermodynamics** states the change in the internal energy of a system is equal to the heat added to the system minus the work being done from the system.
  E IN vs. E Out
- **Law of Energy Conservation** states that energy is always conserved; it cannot be created or destroyed. Energy can be converted from one form into another.
  You can't make something from nothing.

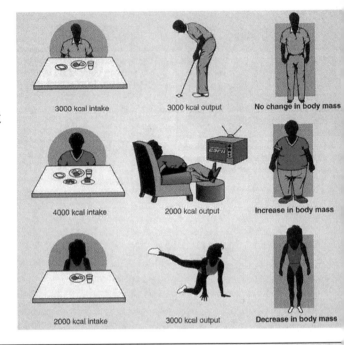

3000 kcal intake   3000 kcal output   No change in body mass

4000 kcal intake   2000 kcal output   Increase in body mass

2000 kcal intake   3000 kcal output   Decrease in body mass

Overcoming the confusion of the causes of Weight Gain
Genetics and Lifestyle variables:

Genetics
Genetics has been used as a limitation for individuals seeking weight management. Taking the science in to account, there is no debate. Calorie intake vs. Calorie expenditure.
Using a card game as an example: Genetics is the hand you are dealt.

Lifestyle
How you play the hand you are dealt.
Hectic Schedules - causing eating on the go or missing meals. You don't plan to fail, you fail to plan.
Stress – This topic is potentially the biggest of them all. The body will lose the ability to burn calories over time do to muscle tissue loss.
Social & Lifestyle Patterns – We center much of our socialization on gathering to eat too much and drink alcohol.
Lack of education - as it relates to nutrition. We buy into a lot of fads and popular myths. We will dispel a few of them later.
Bottom Line:
Your Genetics will determine *how fast* you can lose/gain weight.
Your Lifestyle will ultimately determine if you gain/lose weight.

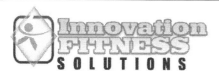

How many Calories should I eat?

*Perform both calculations, average the two and add the multiplier

---

Calculation #1   (The Harris-Benedict Equation)

Males: $66 + (13.7 \times \text{weight in kg}) + (5 \times \text{height in cm}) - (6.8 \times \text{age}) = \text{BMR}$
Females: $655 + (9.6 \times \text{weight in kg}) + (1.7 \times \text{height in cm}) - (4.7 \times \text{age}) = \text{BMR}$

Calculation #2   (The Katch - McArdle Equation)

Male & Female: $370 + (21.6 \times \text{lean body mass in kg}) = \text{BMR}$

*Body composition testing is needed to determine lean body mass
Once you have determined your BMR, you then multiply your BMR by your daily activity caloric burn.

Activity Multiplier:
- ✓ Sedentary = BMR X 1.2 (little or no exercise, desk job)
- ✓ Lightly active = BMR X 1.375 (light exercise/sports 1-3 days/wk)
- ✓ Moderate active = BMR X 1.55 (moderate exercise/sports 3-5 days/wk)
- ✓ Very active = BMR X 1.725 (hard exercise/sports 6-7 days/wk)

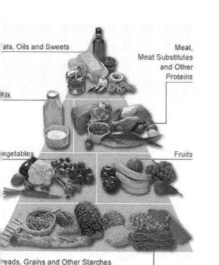

Calculation #1	=
Calculation #2	=
Average	=
Activity	=
Daily Calorie Allotment	=

www.InnovationFitnessSolutions.com

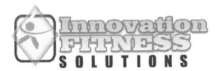

Take charge of your results

The more detailed and consistent and reliable your information is the easier it is to do your calorie detective work if/when a setback arises. To avoid calorie amnesia, jot down everything you consume right away. Start to pay attention to the calorie content of the items you choose by reading food labels and looking up the calorie content of restaurant foods and beverages.

Keep in mind that many beverages contain calories so be sure to count your calorie containing liquids (Teas, Coffees, sports drinks and alcohol). They add up quickly.

Use the internet to learn the calorie content of your favorite and most frequently eaten foods. Humans are creatures of habit, you'll get familiar with the items you eat regularly and measuring will no longer be necessary. The idea is to get educated on how much you eat and to know your "go to" foods.

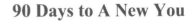

> **Tips on Food Journaling:**
>
> 1. **Write as you go.**
>   As soon as you eat it, ink it.
> 2. **Pre Journal.**
>   Write your planned meals/snacks out the night prior. Use a different color pen to check off or write the differences.
> 3. **Bookend the weekend.**
>   Journal on Friday's and Monday's. This will keep you on track if you have been doing it a while.

The scale never lies long term.
On any given day, the scale can deceive you and your true progress won't be accurately reflected by your weight. This is because body weight can fluctuate on a daily basis due to the amount of fluid we retain. Foods high in sodium, menstrual cycles, certain medications and bowel movements can increase fluid retention and skew your weight.

However, over time the scale tells the whole story. If your weight creeps up after two or three weeks, you've been eating more calories than you're burning. The opposite is also true – if your weight decreases after two to three weeks, you've been eating fewer calories than you're burning. A steady weight indicates the calories you're burning and consuming are equal.

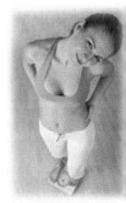

Patience

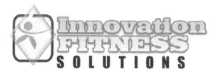

Weight Range:
One suggestion is to not think in terms of Bodyweight. Use a **bodyweight range.**
Weigh yourself for 4 days in a row. Record your highest weight during that time and your lowest weight. You have just found your bodyweight range!
It is usually a 2-4 lb. difference. Use the range to measure your success.

Ex: If you weight fluctuates from 150 lbs to 155 lbs that (150 -155) is your range. Measure your progress off of the range, not the static scale number. It will not be the same from day to day.

Tips for Weighing In
After you have found your starting BW range be sure to weigh yourself at least once a week once you get started.
To minimize fluctuations, follow these tips for weighing in:

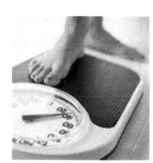

- Wear similar clothing each time
- Use the same scale
- Weigh in at the same time of day
- Maintain similar eating and drinking patterns prior to weighing in
- Weigh in mid-week if you only check your weight weekly.
- Monday weigh-ins tend to be inaccurate because of food choices and eating habits on weekends

Other Ways to Measure Progress
- If you're making progress in at least two of the following areas, you're on the right track:
- Inches lost, Body fat percentage, Clothing size or fit, Energy levels, Positive Mental Attitude

---

Stand while working whenever possible.
Make a list of activities you could do while standing and check them off each time you do them. Some ideas:
- ✓ Talking on the phone
- ✓ Talking to co-workers, family or friends
- ✓ Reading the mail
- ✓ Working on the computer (if you can raise your monitor or laptop without hunching over)
- ✓ Folding laundry
- ✓ Watching TV

Move

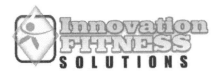

Key Points: Day 1-30

✓ Eat a balanced breakfast when you wake up.

✓ Do not go more than 3 to 4 hours without eating (unless you are sleeping).

✓ Try to eat 3 meals and 1-2 snacks per day.

✓ Eat a snack composed of carbohydrates, protein, and fat within 45 minutes after completing a workout to help repair damaged muscle and replenish muscle glycogen (energy) stores.

✓ Do not save the majority of your calories for one meal – your body cannot handle more than 50% of its calories at one time, and your body will end up storing the food as fat.

✓ Schedule your workouts and movement.

✓ Plan to do something every day that will bring you closer to your goal.

✓ Mentally prepare yourself for setbacks. Be resilient in adversity and determined to find a solution.

✓ Take your Multi Vitamin daily.

✓ Stay Positive and Find a reason to smile often.

✓ Set Goals that are challenging but attainable. Do not set goals you cannot reach and cannot maintain.

✓ Find Non- Gym based activities to do that you enjoy.

✓ Keep in mind that weight loss slows down. Do not expect the same results in Week 6 that you had in Week1.

✓ Don't give up! Don't EVER give up!

Weekly Report Card:

Rate your progress on a 1(Low) – 5(Great) scale.	
Food	
Did you keep your Food Journal?	**Avg # of meals daily?**
Are you planning ahead: ☐	**Meal Timing?**
Avg. H2O Daily: ☐	**Quality of food**:
Sleeping Well: ☐ **Hours:**	**Energy Level:**
Meal Timing: (Hours):	**Speed of Eating**:
Coffee/ Caloric Drinks:	**Alcohol:**
Multi Vitamin:	
Fitness	
Accidental Exercise (Daily):	**Cardio sessions (Week)**:
Exercise Intensity?	**Strength Training Sessions:**
Mental Fitness	**Success:**

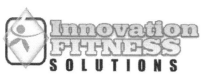
Your Weekly Plan

<u>**I will make these changes to my food this week:**</u>

1.
2.
3.
4.
5.
6.
7.

<u>**I will add these activities to my week:**</u>

1.
2.
3.
4.
5.
6.
7.

<u>**I experienced these successes this week:**</u>

1.
2.
3.
4.
5.
6.
7.

**available for download from www.InnovationFitnessSolutions.com

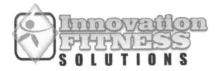

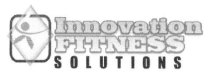

Days 31 – 60 - Physical Activity Changes

"You cannot solve a problem with the same mind that created it."
-Albert Einstein

"No action, no change. Limited action, limited change. Lots of action, change occurs."
-Catherine Pulsifer

Welcome to the second month your total life transformation. Last month we reviewed setting ourselves up for long term success by preparing mentally and arming ourselves with all the necessary tools we'll need. This month we will discuss the physical side to our continued success. Here is a cute little saying I picked up from one of my business associates, it really explains how to attain and maintain long term success:
"Prior Proper Planning Prevents Poor Performance"

There is no doubt that by maintaining your journal you began to realize all of the 'hidden' calories that we consume. It's frustrating that we can beat ourselves up in the gym for 90 minutes to burn a measly 400 -600 calories and then put it all back in to our body with 1.5 glasses of wine. However, with the 'honesty covenant' that we have with ourselves there is no frustration. When we keep a food and exercise journal we have credible, detailed information to aid us in making logical decisions. Remaining logical is of paramount importance. Working out consistently is hard work. Trying to change your body for good is even harder. Every calorie counts and you need to stay focused and detailed and deliberate.

By following the recommendations set last month there was most likely a few things that occurred:
1) You lost a fair amount of weight fairly quickly.
2) Awareness of your habits (good and bad).
3) You found movement to be enjoyable.
4) You dealt with your stress a bit better.
5) You began to feel more energetic and prepared.

Here are the goals for this month:
1. To create a progressive cardiovascular program.
2. To create a progressive resistance training program.
3. To maintain the positive state of mind from last month.
4. To realize that you cannot keep doing the same workout as usual for Fat Loss.
5. To learn Body Basics.

What did you learn about yourself last month?

1.
2.
3.

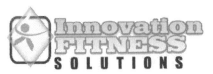

The Workout Plan = Upside down and inside out.

Working out improves your health, fitness and longevity. Initially when you begin a new workout regimen the physiological changes are significant. Your Nervous System is working incredibly hard to figure out how to handle all of these "new, unaccustomed" stimuli that it's experiencing. You end up burning a significant amount of extra calories every day in an attempt to recover from this new experience. The downside is…this does not last. Our body is designed for survival. That means that it is great at conserving and storing energy. This is a true disadvantage to those of us trying to reverse the amount of stored energy that we have. We have seen many people start an exercise plan with Fat Loss as a goal but it turns into an "Anti Weight Gain Plan" because they allow their body to adapt to the plan. The best way to utilize the workout for continual Fat Loss is to change it frequently.

Here are a few items that you need to know. Chances are you have or will experience most of them. The good news is you are not the first person and we know how to deal with it.

A Quick Review:

1. **Bottom line to weigh less:** E (energy) IN vs. E (energy) OUT. If you are attempting to lose weight/fat you need to expend more calories than you consume. If you are not losing weight you are not in a deficit. Stop coming up with reasons or excuses and review your intake in its entirety, then review your exercise plan to insure that you are maximizing your efforts in the gym.

2. **Pay attention to your hunger and hunger cues:** Many people will experience a rise in hunger and appetite as a result of initiating a new workout plan. If this is your case you'll need to make small dietary changes (eat by the clock - not by the stomach, change the P, C, F composition of the meal/snack) to insure that you do not get too hungry and end up overeating.

3. **Nourish your body properly:** Exercise increases the need for nutrients. If you are simultaneously dieting you are in a nutrient deficit. This can begin to ruin your 'metabolism'. Make sure you are taking your daily Multi Vitamin <u>DAILY.</u>

4. **Different Goals require different action plans.** Working out for the goal of Long Term Fat Loss is different in methodology from working out for Fitness and Health. **Efficient body = Lack of Fat Loss Results:** Working out initially burns a significant amount of extra calories. The body strives for "the path of least resistance". This means that it likes to be efficient. This is counter- productive towards any Fat Loss goal. Mentally, you are striving to burn more calories; physically your body is trying to figure out how to burn less…

44

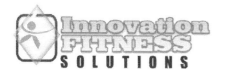

5. **GET OFF THE TREADMILL:** If you are exercising for the same amount of time and at the same intensity on the same machines for more than a month you are allowing the body to become efficient. (S.A.I.D. Principle) This s l o w s fat loss/ calorie burning down.

6. **Kick up your intensity:** Many people never maximize their effort. I am an advocate of coming to the gym frequently. It burns calories, maintains tone, and improves overall health. All of these are great! But, if you are attempting to alter your body composition it takes a bit more than just showing up. An all out effort as frequently as possible will increase your calorie burn. When you don't have it to give show up anyway and work out. When you do have that 'tweaked' mental state - use it! Lift heavier, run faster, jump higher, do more repetitions. As NIKE says: Just Do IT! RIGHT NOW!

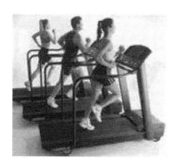 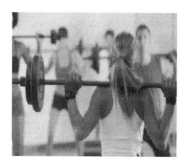

The Actual Workout:

I like to name my workouts. It gives a sense of ownership. Plus, workout intensity is just as much of mental strength as it is physical strength. You have got to get 'geared up' to workout hard and burn calories. A few names that I use frequently: Achievement, Personal Best, No Excuses, Assault, No Nonsense, Do It, Do It Again!, I will do this, I can and will do more, 1 more!… I think about the name and what workout images it conjures up. Generally, if you're driving over to the gym and visualizing the name and the workout you will improve your mental state. The "I am going to the gym and working out because I have to" mentality morphs into "I am going to rip the doors off of this place". Bottom line is if the goal is fat loss, increasing your intensity burns more calories per minute and that improves the effectiveness of your workouts. All these strategies are geared towards maximizing your time. To get the most form your workouts you have got to be prepared mentally and physically for them. A few alterations to get you on the right track:

1. **Lift heavier.** Like I previously mentioned with intensity you'll get out of your comfort zone and produce different results. Ladies, don't worry about "getting big". It takes a lot more than just lifting a little heavier to produce dramatic gains in musculature.

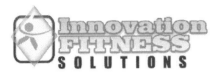

2. **Lift Lighter and do more repetitions.** Just the opposite of the above. If you are used to training with heavier weights then decrease your weight by 15-20% and do as many repetitions as possible. Your body will respond very differently.

3. **Circuit train.** Perform a strength training move followed by a cardio move for 30 sec – 1 min and don't stop. If you do a chest press, then do a ladder drill. You won't give your body a chance to slow down and you'll end up burning more calories in less time.

4. **Superset.** Pick two or three exercises in a row. Similar to above do them all in succession without rest. Try not to make them all for the same body part. You'll end up burning a substantial amount of calories but not overdoing and creating unwanted soreness in any one area.

5. **Choose a different cardio machine** every two weeks and vow to kick your own butt every time. Cardio machines are where I see many people go wrong. They get on a treadmill, get really good at walking/jogging/running on the treadmill and never, ever leave. The body adapts to everything. Pick something else to boost your calorie burning.

6. **Sleep**. You don't get enough. Get more. It aids in recovery and will reenergize you for your big workout tomorrow. We suggest 6-8 hours a night consistently. We realize that for many of you this is an issue. You must find new relaxations strategies (Darker room, turn the T.V. off, read) to prepare you to sleep quicker. Studies have shown that overtired people tend to eat more food too. This certainly will not aid your efforts.

7. **Do partner training** with a personal trainer. This one act overcomes many obstacles. It sets an appointment that you'll keep because not only are you paying for it but someone else is counting on you to show up. We skip too many workouts for not good enough reasons. This also makes training more affordable and fun.

8. **Add tools and toys** to spice things up. Stability balls, tubing, bands, cables all add new and different challenges to a stale routine. You'll work balance, strength, coordination and endurance all

9. **Surprise Exercise:** Do not under any circumstance let me see you looking for the closest parking space to the front door of the gym unless you have 3 + kids, a gym bag, a stroller and a broken foot.

10. **Make your 3+ kids a workout**. Push-ups, sit-up and running challenges against your kids are a ton of fun! They like it and you need it! Plus you'll be laughing a lot and that will help to "tone" your stomach. Make your goal to tire them out!

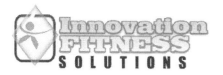

Kids Ctd... Also, if they are young use them as weights for no other reason than to move. Lift them up and do 10 -20 squats and lunges.

11. **Take a Group Fitness Class** that you have not tried before. You will find that when you work out with others you will work harder for longer. You will burn more calories and have more fun.

12. **Interval Bursts** You've probably heard about the benefits of interval training, but just keep in mind that a true "fat burning interval" shouldn't last more than 10 – 30 seconds and needs to be ALL OUT. Advanced exercisers may be able to handle a full minute, but that's about it.

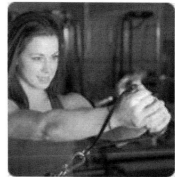

13. **Purchase home workout equipment**. Go to your local sporting goods store and purchase a set or two of lightweight dumbbells, a jump rope, a piece of exercise tubing and store it in plain sight. Set your phone alarm or computer calendar to go off every hour or two, get up go for a 5 minute stroll and spend 5 minutes lifting weights. You'll burn an extra 100-200 calories daily and increase your "tone". Add up the calories through the course of a year and really be impressed. Perform 2-3 sets whenever you pass by the equipment. Time yourself for 1 minute and do the exercise continually or perform a set of 15-20 repetitions, wait one minute and do it again.

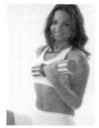

    a. Push-ups
    b. Sit-ups/Crunches
    c. Squats
    d. Lunges
    e. Bicep Curls
    f. Rowing
    g. Side Bends and Twists

14. **Stand while working whenever possible**. Spend some time today examining how you spend your time, whether at work or at home. If you spend much of your time sitting, give your body a break by standing up as much as possible. Make a list of activities you could do while standing and check them off each time you do them. Some ideas:
    a. Talking on the phone
    b. Talking to co-workers, family or friends
    c. Reading the mail
    d. Working on the computer (if you can raise your monitor or laptop without hunching over)
    e. Folding laundry or watching TV

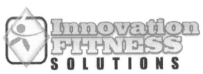

15. **Interval Bursts** You've probably heard about the benefits of interval training, but just keep in mind that a true "fat burning interval" shouldn't last more than 10 – 30 seconds and needs to be ALL OUT. Advanced exercisers may be able to handle a full minute, but that's about it.

16. **High Intensity Training** should be done with some type of resistance (body weight, bands, free weights, kettlebells, etc) and provide a serious stimulus to your body. Also, these workouts shouldn't last for more than 20 – 40 minutes.

17. **Squats.** Yes, squats… if you didn't do anything else in your entire workout except squats you would still turn your body into a fat burning furnace! Unfortunately, most people don't think they can squat until they realize that every time they go to sit down they're squatting. Squatting is NOT bad for your knees… only squatting improperly is.

18. **Frontal and Transverse Plane Movements**
During every day activities we typically we move our bodies forwards and backwards (sagital plane). We feel comfortable doing this and as a result our workouts reflect this one movement as well… So, one trick is to add side-to-side (frontal plane) and rotational movements (transverse plane) into your exercise program. This provides a "shock" and new stimulus to the body and will give your metabolism a nice boost!

19. **Metabolic Boost Workouts**: INTENSITY
In order to change your body you need to give your body a reason to change. That doesn't mean beating yourself up or using poor form to lift heavy weights, but you *will* need to push your comfort zone. Unless you do something to make your body keep up, it's happy to remain the same way it currently is.

20. **Stretch in the shower.** Extend your shower time by 5 minutes and do a few stretches for your back, some twisting motions and for your hips. You will get an added bonus on top of the flexibility increase because it will most likely improve your mood too.

21. **Take a Group Exercise Class or Martial arts class.** It will provide a boost to your workout because there will be others there to motivate you and every class is different so it will prevent boredom. Studies show people are 40% more likely to stick to an exercise program when they workout in groups.

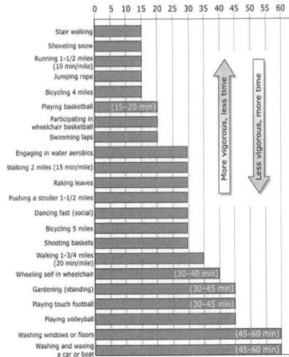

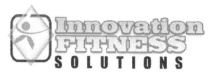

Cardiovascular Exercise Plans

| 12 Week Cardiovascular Program (Beginner – Intermediate Exerciser) |

Week 1	Cross trainer	3 times per week	Level 4-5 Intensity	20-30 Minutes
Week 2	Cross trainer	3 times per week	Level 4-5 Intensity	20-30 Minutes
Week 3	Treadmill	3 times per week	Level 4-5 Intensity	20-30 Minutes
Week 4	Treadmill	3 times per week	Level 5-6 Intensity	30-40 Minutes
Week 5	Stairmaster	4 times per week	Level 5-6 Intensity	30-40 Minutes
Week 6	Stairmaster	4 times per week	Level 5-6 Intensity	30-40 Minutes
Week 7	Cross trainer 2	4 times per week	Level 5-6 Intensity	30-40 Minutes
Week 8	Cross trainer 2	4 times per week	Level 6-7 Intensity	30-40 Minutes
Week 9	Treadmill	5 times per week	Level 6-7 Intensity	30-40 Minutes
Week 10	Treadmill	5 times per week	Level 6-7 Intensity	40-50 Minutes
Week 11	Cross trainer 1	5 times per week	Level 8 Intensity	40-50 Minutes
Week 12	Cross trainer 1	5 times per week	Level 8 Intensity	40-50 Minutes

* Do not hold handrails while exercising. Maintain an upright posture to burn more Cal.

**We highly recommend the use of a heart rate watch to monitor intensity.

***All of your weight cannot be lost at once. Follow your protocols for success.

**** A maintenance phase of 2-4 weeks should follow this protocol.

Park in the furthest parking space from the door
Each time you go somewhere today, make it a point to park as far from the door as you can to add more walking to your daily routine.

49

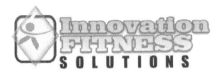

12 Week Cardiovascular Program (Intermediate/Advanced Cross training)				
Week 1	Cross trainer	4 times per week	Level 5 Intensity	30 Minutes
Week 2	Treadmill	4 times per week	Level 5 Intensity	30 Minutes
Week 3	Cross trainer/ Treadmill	4 times per week	Level 4-5 Intensity	20 Minutes 20 Minutes
Week 4	Cross trainer/ Treadmill	4 times per week	Level 5-6 Intensity Level 7 Intensity	25 Minutes 15 Minutes
Week 5	Stairmaster	5 times per week	Level 5-6 Intensity	40 Minutes
Week 6	Cross trainer 2	5 times per week	Level 5-6 Intensity	40 Minutes
Week 7	Stairmaster/ Cross trainer 2	5 times per week	Level 5-6 Intensity Level 7 Intensity	25 Minutes 15 Minutes
Week 8	Stairmaster/ Cross trainer 2	5 times per week	Level 6-7 Intensity Level 7 Intensity	20 Minutes 20 Minutes
Week 9	Treadmill	5 times per week	Level 6-7 Intensity	30-40 Minutes
Week 10	Cross trainer 1	5 times per week	Level 6-7 Intensity	40-50 Minutes
Week 11	Treadmill/ Cross trainer 1	5 times per week	Level 8 Intensity	25 Minutes 25 Minutes
Week 12	Treadmill/ Cross trainer 1	5 times per week	Level 8 Intensity	20 Minutes 30 Minutes

Interval Training for Beginners - Level 1

The following workout is a beginner interval workout lasting 21 minutes.
Interval workouts involve alternating higher intensity exercise with low intensity recovery periods.
Interval workouts involve alternating higher intensity exercise with low intensity recovery periods.
By adding higher intensity intervals, you can build endurance and burn more calories.
The workout is shown using a treadmill with changes in speed and incline, but you can use any machine of your choice or take the workout outside.

Workout Instructions
For each 'work set', use the settings on your machine (incline, speed, resistance, ramps, etc.) to increase intensity.
You should be working out of your comfort zone, but not so hard that you feel dizzy or lightheaded.
For each 'rest set', lower those same settings until you're back to a moderate pace.
You should be completely recovered before the next work set.

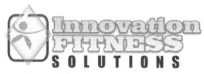

*Modify according to your fitness level.

The RPE levels listed (Rate of <u>Perceived Exertion</u>) help you keep track of your intensity on a scale of 1 - 10. During rest sets, stay around 4-5 RPE. During work sets, stay around 6-7 RPE. There isn't a huge difference between the work and rest sets, you simply want to work a little harder during the work sets.

Interval	Beginner Workout 1 - 21 Minutes
Warm up	5 Minutes: RPE 3-4: *Easy pace
Rest Set	3 Minutes: RPE 5: Increase speed from warm up and increase incline 1%. Keep a moderate pace.
Work Set	1 Minute: RPE 6 - Increase incline 1-3% to raise the intensity level. You should be working harder!
Rest Set	3 Minutes: RPE 5 - Decrease speed and incline to lower your heart rate back to a comfortable level
Work Set	1 Minute: RPE 6 - Increase speed 3-5 increments and increase incline 1-2% to raise intensity.
Rest Set	3 Minutes: RPE 5 - Decrease speed and incline to lower your heart rate back to a comfortable level
Cool down	5 Minutes: RPE 3-5 - Decrease speed/incline to lower your heart rate back to a comfortable level and cool down

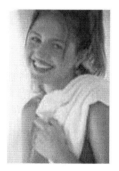
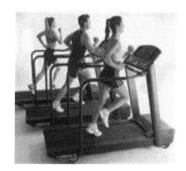

Cardio Gym Workouts: 30-Minute Treadmill Intervals – Boredom Buster

This cardio workout will help you bust boredom and burn calories by changing your speed, resistance and/or incline throughout the workout. You'll alternate intensity intervals where you'll work at a high intensity along with recovery intervals. Increase or decrease the speed and/or duration of each interval according to your fitness level and use the <u>Perceived Exertion Scale</u> to determine how hard you're working. The speeds and inclines listed are only suggestions, please modify as needed.

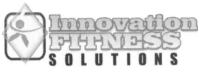

Time	Intensity/Speed	Incline	Perceived Exertion
5 min.	3.0 mph - warm-up	1%	Level 2-3
5 min.	3.5 - 4.5 - walk/slow jog	1%	Level 4
1 min	5.0 - 5.5 - speed walk/run	2%	Level 6
2 min	4.0 - 5.0 - walk/slow jog	0%	Level 4
1 min	5.0 - 5.5 - speed walk/ run	2%	Level 6-7
2 min	4.0 - 5.0 - walk/slow jog	0%	Level 4
1 min	5.3 - 5.7 - speed walk/run	1-2%	Level 7
2 min	4.0 - 5.0 - walk/ slow jog	0%	Level 4
1 min	Walk or run as fast as you can	1-2%	Level 7-8
2 min	4.0 - 5.0 - walk/ slow jog	0%	Level 4
5 min	3.0 - 4.0	0%	Level 3

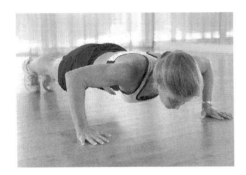

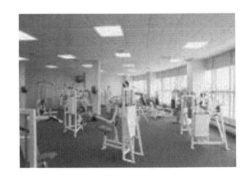

Resistance Training

Resistance training is a key to altering your appearance and burning calories. Many people mistakenly assume that dieting and/or cardiovascular work is all it will take to look the way that they want to. This is false.

- ✓ Resistance training adds "tone" to your appearance. It is what gives you the athletic look that most desire.
- ✓ It burns more calories per minute than most cardiovascular exercise.
- ✓ It burns calories for an extended period after the actual workout.
- ✓ It may improve bone mineral density.
- ✓ It allows you to eat more food.

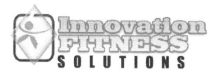

Workout Notes: In the first 2 weeks of the program, do the circuit twice. Move from exercise to exercise with no more than 30 seconds of rest in between. When you complete one circuit, rest for 1 to 2 minutes and complete the second circuit.

After the first 2 weeks, when you've become comfortable doing two complete circuits during a workout, increase your workload to three circuits per workout. In every exercise, use a weight that you can handle comfortably for the number of repetitions noted. When that becomes too easy, increase the weight on each set by 10 percent.

MONDAY

Total-Body Strength Training Workout - Complete one set of each abs exercise*, then complete the rest of the circuit twice.

Exercise	Repetitions	Rest	Sets
Traditional Crunch*	12-15		1
Bent-Leg Knee Raise*	12-15		1
Oblique V-Up*	10 each side		1
Bridge*	1 or 2		1
Back Extensions*	12-15		1
Squats	10-12	30 seconds	2
Bench Press	10	30 seconds	2
Pulldown	10	30 seconds	2
Military Press	10	30 seconds	2
Side Lunges	10 each side	30 seconds	2
Triceps Pushdown	10-12	30 seconds	2
Leg Extension	10-12	30 seconds	2
Biceps Curl	10	30 seconds	2
Leg Curl	10-12	30 seconds	2

WEDNESDAY

Total-Body Strength Training Workout with Abs Emphasis. Complete one set of each abs exercise*, then complete the rest of the circuit twice.

Exercise	Repetitions	Rest	Sets
Standing Crunch *	12-15		1
Pulse Up *	12		1
Saxon Side Bend *	6-10 each side		1
Side Bridge*	1 or 2		1
Back Extensions*	12-15		1
Squats	10-12	30 seconds	2
Bench Press	10	30 seconds	2
Pulldown	10	30 seconds	2
Military Press	10	30 seconds	2
Twist Lunge	10 each side	30 seconds	2
Triceps Pushdown	10-12	30 seconds	2
Leg Extension	10-12	30 seconds	2
Biceps Curl	10	30 seconds	2

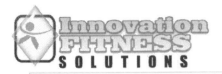

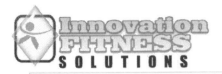

90 Days to A New You

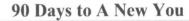

FRIDAY

Total-Body Strength Training Workout with Leg Emphasis. Repeat entire circuit twice.

Exercise	Repetitions	Rest	Sets
Squats	10-12	30 seconds	2
Bench Press	10	30 seconds	2
Pulldown	10	30 seconds	2
Traveling Lunge	10-12 each leg	30 seconds	2
Military Press	10	30 seconds	2
Push Ups	10	30 seconds	2
Step-Up	10-12 each leg	30 seconds	2
Triceps Pushdown	10-12	30 seconds	2
Leg Extension	10-12	30 seconds	2
Biceps Curl	10	30 seconds	2
Leg Curl	10-12	30 seconds	2

Basic Exercise Descriptions

Squat

Hold a barbell with an overhand grip so that it rests comfortably on your upper back. Set your feet shoulder-width apart, and keep your knees slightly bent, back straight, and eyes focused straight ahead. Slowly lower your body as if you were sitting back into a chair, keeping your back in its natural alignment and your lower legs nearly perpendicular to the floor. When your thighs are parallel to the floor, pause, then return to the starting position.

Home variation: Same, but with one dumbbell in each hand, your palms facing your outer thighs.

Variations: Split Stance Squat/Lunge. Stagger your feet so one foot is behind the body and one foot ahead.

Bench Press

Lie on your back on a flat bench with your feet on the floor. Grab the barbell with an overhand grip, your hands just beyond shoulder-width apart. Lift the bar off the uprights, and hold it at arm's length over your chest. Slowly lower the bar to your chest. Pause, and then push the bar back to the starting position.

Home variation: Just do standard Pushups: Get in a Pushup position with your hands about shoulder-width apart. Bend at the elbows while keeping your back straight, until your chin almost touches the floor, and then push back up.

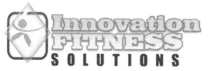

Pulldown

Stand facing a lat pulldown machine. Grasp the bar with an overhand grip that's 4 to 6 inches wider than your shoulders. Sit on the seat, letting the resistance of the bar extend your arms above your head. When you're in position, pull the bar down until it is level with your nose. Hold this position for a second, and then return to the starting position.

Home variation: Bent-Over Row. Stand with your knees slightly bent and shoulder-width apart. Bend over so that your back is almost parallel to the floor. Holding a dumbbell in each hand let your arms hang toward the floor. With your palms facing in, pull the dumbbells toward you until they touch the outside of your chest. Pause, and then return to the starting position.

Military Press

Sitting on an exercise bench, hold a barbell at shoulder height with your hands shoulder-width apart. Press the weight straight overhead so that your arms are almost fully extended, hold for a count of one, and then bring it down to the front of your shoulders. Repeat.

Home variation: Sitting on a sturdy chair instead of a bench, hold one dumbbell in each hand, about level with your ears. Push the dumbbells straight overhead so that your arms are almost fully extended, hold for a count of one, then return to the starting position.

Triceps Pushdown

While standing, grip a bar attached to a high pulley cable or lat machine with your hands about 6 inches apart. With your elbows tucked against your sides, bring the bar down until it is directly in front of you. With your forearms parallel to the floor (the starting position), push the bar down until your arms are extended straight down with the bar near your thighs. Don't lock your elbows. Return to the starting position.

Home variation: Triceps Kickback. Stand with your knees slightly bent and shoulder-width apart. Bend over so that your back is almost parallel to the ground. Bend your elbows to about 90-degree angles, raising them to just above the level of your back. This is the starting position. Extend your forearms backward, keeping your upper arms stationary. When they're fully extended, your arms should be parallel to the ground. Pause, and then return to the starting position.

Leg Extension

Sitting on a leg extension machine with your feet under the footpads, lean back slightly, and lift the pads with your feet until your legs are extended.

Home variation: Squat Against the Wall. Stand with your back flat against a wall. Squat down so that your thighs are parallel to the ground. Hold that position for as long as you can. That consists of one set. Aim for 20 seconds to start, and work your way up to 45 seconds.

Biceps Curl

Stand while holding a barbell in front of you, palms facing out, with your hands shoulder-width apart and your arms hanging in front of you. Curl the weight toward your shoulders, hold for a second, and then return to the starting position. Home variation: Same, only use a set of dumbbells instead.

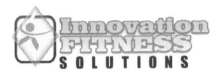

Leg Curl

Lie face down on a leg curl machine, and hook your ankles under the padded bar. Keeping your stomach and pelvis against the bench, slowly raise your feet toward your butt, curling up the weight. Come up so that your feet nearly touch your butt, and slowly return to the starting position.
Home variation: Lie down with your stomach on the floor. Put a light dumbbell between your feet (so that the top end of the dumbbell rests on the bottom of your feet). Squeeze your feet together, and curl them up toward your butt.

Traveling Lunge

Rest a barbell across your upper back. Stand, with your feet hip-width apart, at one end of the room; you need room to walk about 20 steps. Step forward with your left foot, and lower your body so that your left thigh is parallel to the floor and your right thigh is perpendicular to the floor (your right knee should bend and almost touch the floor). Stand and bring your right foot up next to your left, then repeat with the right leg lunging forward.
Home variation: Use dumbbells, holding one in each hand with your arms at your sides. If you don't have enough space, do the move in one place, alternating your lead foot with each lunge.

Step-Up

Use a step or bench that's 18 inches off the ground. Place your left foot on the step so that your knee is bent at 90 degrees. Your knee should not advance past the toes of your left foot. Push off with your left foot, and bring your right foot onto the step, keeping your back straight. Now step down with the left foot, followed by the right. Alternate the leading foot, or do all of the repetitions leading with one foot and then alternating. Once you're comfortable, add dumbbells.
Home variation: Same, only use a staircase instead of a step (if you don't have one).

Saxon Side Bend

Hold a pair of lightweight dumbbells over your head, in line with your shoulders, with your elbows slightly bent. Keep your back straight, and slowly bend directly to your left side as far as possible without twisting your upper body. Pause, return to an upright position, then bend to your right side as far as possible. 6 - 10 reps on each side, no rest between sets

Side Bridge

Lie on your nondominant side. Support your weight with that forearm and the outside edge of that foot. Your body should form a straight line from head to ankles. Pull your abs in as far as you can, and hold this position for 10 to 30 seconds, breathing steadily. Relax. If you can do 30 seconds, do one repetition. If not, try for any combination of reps that gets you up to 30 seconds. Repeat on your other side. 1 - 2 reps on each side, no rest between sets

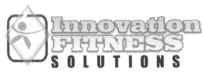

Days 31 – 60 Articles: Exercise

Exercise or movement has a number of health and longevity benefits. It has long been known that exercise is a key factor in improving or maintaining the following:

- ✓ *Cardiovascular health*
- ✓ *Increasing Bone Mineral Density*
- ✓ *Increasing Metabolism (rate the body burns calories)*
- ✓ *Maintaining Muscle Tone*
- ✓ *Increasing Strength and Stamina*
- ✓ *Improving Activities of Daily Living*
- ✓ *Maintaining Ideal Bodyweight*
- ✓ *Burns Calories*
- ✓ *Allows you to eat more food*

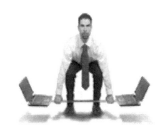

*The average adult loses a half pound of muscle tissue annually while gaining 1.5 pounds of body fat (sarcopenia). This results in a loss of "tone" and a loss in the ability to burn stored calories (body fat) for fuel. The numbers may be a bit deceiving if you were measuring on a scale as it would only be a 1 pound total weight gain. In reality, however, the composition/ *weight shift* of the body has changed a full 2 pounds. Many believe that this change in body composition or weight shift is due to an increasingly sedentary environment either at work and/or home. It becomes imperative to find ways and reasons to move more throughout the day.

Moderate Physical Activity *Source: Adapted from the 2005 DGAC Report*	Approximate Calories/Hr for a 154 lb Person[a]
Hiking	370
Light gardening/yard work	330
Dancing	330
Golf (walking and carrying clubs)	330
Bicycling (<10 mph)	290
Walking (3.5 mph)	280
Weight lifting (general light workout)	220
Vigorous Physical Activity	Approximate Calories/Hr for a 154 lb Person[a]
Running/jogging (5 mph)	590
Bicycling (>10 mph)	590
Swimming (slow freestyle laps)	510
Aerobics	480
Walking (4.5 mph)	460
Heavy yard work (chopping wood)	440
Weight Lifting (Vigorous)	440
Basketball	440

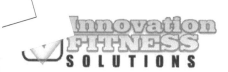

15 ways to add "Surprise Exercise" into your day

There are 3500 calories in 1 lb. of Body fat. Add these in to your day to increase calorie expenditure and quicken the pace that your fat melts off! Choose 2-3 of these a week and add up the calorie burn!

1. ***Balance Booster.*** While you brush your teeth, alternate standing on one leg as you move the toothbrush from one area of the mouth to another (every 30 seconds). This will help develop your core muscles and may even be good for your coordination. **Burns 10 Calories**

2. ***Be a Ballerina.*** As your coffee drips, stand sideways, put one hand on the counter, and lift the outside leg straight out in front of you, keeping it extended. With upper body straight, hold for a few seconds and move it to the side; hold and extend it behind you. Do five to ten times on each leg. Tones outer thighs, hip flexors and quadriceps. **Burns 10 Calories**

3. ***Tone in Traffic.*** Use the time spent bumper-to-bumper to develop derriere. These are called isotonic exercises. Squeeze your buns each time you tap the brake, holding for 10 seconds. Shoot for 10 to 15 squeezes a trip. **Burns 10 Calories**

4. ***Extra Squats.*** A few times a day, while at your desk, pretend you are going to sit but do not and keep your arm out in front of you. Repeat the motion throughout the day. This helps to strengthen your legs, stomach and butt. **Burns 15 Calories**

5. ***Stand in the place that you work.*** Every time you reach for the phone, stand up and walk in place. Studies by the Mayo Clinic have shown that people who are overweight sit on average two and a half hours more per day than their thinner counterparts. **Burns 50 Calories**

6. ***Wall Push-Ups.*** Place hands wide at shoulder height against the wall. Take a couple of steps back so your body is at a slight angle and your weight is on your toes, and do three sets of 10 push-ups. This strengthens the chest and triceps. **Burns 10 Calories**

7. ***Chair Workouts.*** *Dips*: If your chair has wheels, place it against your desk or the wall. Facing forward, place palms on the front edge of the seat with knees bent at a right angle. Lower butt toward the floor; raise and repeat for two sets of 10. This will tone your triceps.
   Lifts: Sitting in a chair with your back straight and your feet on the floor, squeeze knees together and gently bring them toward your chest. Do two sets of ten. This will strengthen your abdominals. ***Burns 10 Calories each***
   Body Pulls: Sitting in a chair with your back straight and your feet on the floor, move your body (and chair) forward by pulling your feet under the chair. **Burns 10 Calories**

8. ***Make an Extra Trip.*** While lugging items upstairs; take one item at a time. After each trip, stop and stand on the bottom step and do calf raises for 8 to 12 reps. **Burns 10 Calories** (per trip)

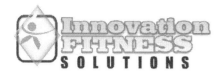

9. ***Strengthen at the Pump.*** Instead of dreading pumping your own gas think of it as an opportunity to improve the strength of your calves. With one hand on your car, stand on the balls of your feet and slowly rise up and down for as long as it takes you to fill your tank. It can be as much as 50 raises if you drive an SUV! **Burns 10 Calories**

10. ***Take the Stairs*** for just two minutes, five days a week, gives you the same calorie-burning results as a 20-minute walk. Now talk about time efficiency. **Burns 120 Calories**

11. ***Commercial Crunches.*** The typical 30-minute TV show has eight minutes of commercials. Every time an ad comes on crunch until the show comes back on; you should reach 100-150 sit-ups or so. Works your stomach muscles. **Burns 25 Calories**

12. ***Lift Those Hips.*** Before you go to sleep at night and get cozy under the blanket, lie on your back on the floor with your legs up on the edge of the bed or a chair. Slowly bend your knees, lifting your hips off the floor. Hold for five seconds, relax and repeat 10 to 12 times. This will firm up your hamstrings and core. **Burns 10 Calories**

13. ***Move It or Lose It!*** You think weekend sports are just for kids? Think again. After every quarter of your kid's soccer or basketball game or after every 2 baseball innings, get up from the bleachers and take a lap around the gym or field. Four or five times around a typical one is about a mile. **Burns 75 Calories**

14. ***Quality Time.*** Spend 30 minutes tossing a ball or Frisbee with your child. (and the time spent is priceless) **Burns 90 Calories**

15. **Mirror, Mirror on the Wall.** Every time you pass a mirror tighten your stomach (make room in your pants) and tighten your butt. Hold this for as long as possible. Tones you stomach and butt. **Burns 5 calories**

> If you have to miss a workout, simply increase your daily activities.
> Wear a Pedometer to challenge yourself (10,000 steps daily).

> Plan meals and workouts by keeping in mind the demands you'll have on your schedule that day.
> Know where you can get a meal that fits your needs.

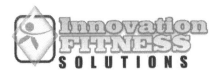

Key Points: Day 31-60

- ✓ Do not go more than 3 to 4 hours without eating (unless you are sleeping).
- ✓ Constantly altering your workouts are essential to maximizing them.
- ✓ Training for the goal of Fat Loss comes down to preserving Lean Tissues and burning as many calories daily as possible!
- ✓ Strength Training is imperative as it maintains your Muscle Tissue (Calorie Burning Machinery).
- ✓ Schedule your workouts and movement.
- ✓ Plan to do something every day that will bring you closer to your goal.
- ✓ Cardiovascular workouts must be altered frequently to avoid adapting to them and minimizing calories burn.
- ✓ Take your Multi Vitamin daily.
- ✓ Stay Positive and Find a reason to smile often.
- ✓ Set Goals that are challenging but attainable.
- ✓ Find Non- Gym based activities to do that you enjoy.
- ✓ Add new machines, exercises and training methods that you have not done before. Your body will respond by burning more calories for a short period.
- ✓ Don't give up! Don't EVER give up!

Weekly Report Card: Day 31-60

Rate your progress on a 1(Low) – 5(Great) scale.

Food

Did you keep your Food Journal?	**Avg # of meals daily?**
Are you planning ahead: ☐	**Meal Timing?**
Avg. H2O Daily: ☐	**Quality of food**:
Sleeping Well: ☐ **Hours:**	**Energy Level:**
Meal Timing: (Hours):	**Speed of Eating:**
Coffee/ Caloric Drinks:	**Alcohol:**
Multi Vitamin:	

Fitness

Accidental Exercise (Daily):	**Cardio sessions (Week):**
Exercise Intensity?	**Strength Training Sessions:**

## Mental Fitness	## Success:
Motivation Level:	**Weight Loss:**
Did you read?	**Inches Lost:**

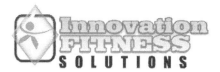

Day 61 – 90
From General Habit Changes to Specific Actions

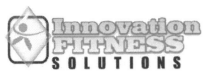

Days 61 – 90 From General Habit Changes to Specific Actions

By following the recommendations set last month there was most likely a few things that occurred:
1) Your weight loss was still decent and you lost a significant amount of inches.
2) Awareness of your habits (good and bad).
3) You found new exercises that challenged you and kept your body changing.
4) You dealt with your stress a bit better.
5) You feel like you're getting in to better shape.

What did you learn about yourself last month?
1
2
3

Here are the goals for this month:
1) To create a plan for realizing and overcoming setbacks.
2) To stay motivated even while some of our progress/measurement methods stall.
3) To maintain the positive state of mind from last month.
4) To take advantage of more specific methods to maximize metabolism...
5) To focus on a plan for 90 days and beyond.

Day 61: Preparing for and overcoming setbacks in your weight loss and motivation
During the first month of this Transformation you most likely had excellent, rapid success without much effort. The second month brought continued success at a good pace but more strategies needed to be utilized. This period you should expect that results will slow down more. We will take a look at why your body HAS to slow down and/or almost stop achieving rapid results and how to alter your Transformation Program to continue your success. The New Habits that have been forming are beginning to feel natural, you are feeling more energetic, your clothing is fitting differently and the mirror is speaking differently to you. Your confidence is really starting to shine through and you are feeling really strong and in shape.
Congratulations.

Take a few minutes and list what you have succeeded at and what remains for you to conquer...
What actions are you taking that are helping you reach your goals? What actions are preventing you from success?

Conquered:	Left to Conquer:
1)	1)
2)	2)
3)	3)
4)	4)
5)	5)

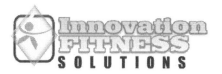

You have accepted TOTAL SELF RESPONSIBILITY. This means that you are in CONTROL. You are aware that you control how much you eat or do not eat. You control how much you move or do not move. You control your environment, it does not control you. You notice that when you have been consistent with your exercise and your eating habits your body reacts positively. You also noticed that if you lose focus for a few days or a week that your body and your mind tend to not go along with what changes you desire…

Successful people do not give up, and you did not. We understand that setbacks are just part of the process and we learn to accept them and continue moving forward. We continue to grow and expand our concept of who we are and our ownership of our body. Towards the end of this month you will begin to be tested for your resiliency, your dedication and your commitment to The New You.

Question: Are you a New You? or the Old You in a temporary new body? Only you know for sure.

"If one advances confidently in the direction of his dreams, and endeavors to live the life which he has imagined, he will meet with success unexpected in common hours." –Thoreau

"Persistence and Determination alone are omnipotent." – Calvin Coolidge

"Change your beliefs and you change your behaviors. Change your behaviors and you change your results. Change your results and you change your life." – Lisa Jimenez

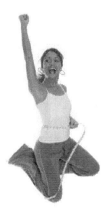

Total Self Responsibility

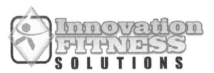

Preparing to Deal with Plateaus and Setbacks

Working with so many clients has made me adeptly aware of the different ways that people deal with setbacks. I have seen many people just give up and contrary to that I have seen many others work through plateaus by doing more and more work or eating less and less. The answer lies somewhere in between.

Plateaus and Setbacks are a natural part of any Weight Loss, Fitness or life process, so you will experience them, the key is to recognize them, understand them and implement the necessary tools to overcome them when you do.
Please do not confuse a Plateau and a Setback. A setback is more mental and behavioral. A plateau is your body physically adjusting to your new activity and your new habits.

Recovering from Setbacks

A setback occurs when we deviate from our planned route. A setback is when we have a food attack or miss workouts or over indulge on desserts and then mentally beat ourselves up for having done so. One of the best ways I know of to get back to "center" is with a list of five Acts of Kindness you will do for yourself (and/or others) when you have a temporary relapse of overeating or an attack on food.

The point is to change the motivation to eat or mentally beat yourself up and return to valuing yourself and your accomplishments. In making your list, think of what will help you stay focused and kind to yourself for longer periods in the future. Perhaps making one of those acts a review of your successes might be helpful to you or a reminder that your clothes are fitting differently and the times that you have felt your confidence boost.

My 5 ways to be kind to myself after a setback:

1.
2.
3.
4.
5.

Setbacks happen to everyone but they do not have to end your quest for success. Successful people find ways to return to positivity quickly and do not dwell on their mistakes. They learn from them and make simple plans for not repeating the same missteps.

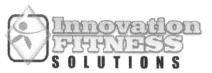

Plateaus are tricky.

Plateaus are extremely frustrating, and what's even more frustrating is not having the tools to Break Through them. A Plateau occurs when your body has found a way to reorganize itself to burn just as many calories as you are consuming even with the presence of exercise and dieting. This is a naturally occurring process and is actually essential to survival. Plateaus happen in all aspects of life, nothing can progress at the same pace forever. Sometimes, you just must slow down; take a strategic break, reorganize and then restart.

An example of a non fitness plateau might be to take a look at the growth of a child, children grow like weeds until their teen years and then continue (slower) well into their twenties. Then, slowly over time they begin to decline in the pace of their vertical growth until by age 25 stop completely. They all possess moments of progression followed by moments of maintenance. Accepting that plateaus will happen is part of the process. With exercise and fitness it is no different.

The body strives for consistency and maintenance. Since your goal is to lose fat, it is important to be able to "trick" the body in order to veer away from a static weight. Oftentimes the process is a difficult one, with multiple starts and stops. It is essential to find areas of progress even if there is no weight loss. Recall form the introduction that everything works, and then it stops working. The key to overcoming plateaus is strategy, planning and consistency.

Recognizing a Plateau:
A plateau can be recognized when your body weight or body fat has not changed after a 1 month period of activity and/or dieting. Initially a plateau manipulation is easy to implement and simple to restart progress. However, an extended plateau is more difficult and tricky. An extended plateau occurs when you have been active in a Transformation Program for multiple months and even after you have manipulated the body by decreasing calorie intake or increasing calorie expenditure multiple times, there still is no change in your weight/fat.

First, we will take a look at how to AVOID plateaus for as long as possible and then we will decide the best Plan of Action for when a Plateau is present.

Weight Loss Plateaus: What's the Cause?

Weight loss plateaus are typically caused by one of two things (sometimes, it's both):

1. A metabolic adaptation to your current diet and exercise regimen
2. Accumulated changes in your existing exercise and eating routine that are causing you to eat more or burn less calories with exercise, even though you aren't aware of it.

65

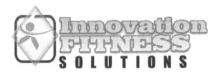
> **What is this metabolic adaptation all about?**
>
> All biological systems have a preference for "homeostasis". Homeostasis is really just a fancy scientific word that describes the body's preference for "staying the same" or "Body Balnace".

Avoiding a Plateau

Initially when you embark on a weight loss plan, you establish a calorie deficit by lowering your caloric intake, increasing your physical activity, or combining both. This calorie deficit is what leads to weight loss. Eventually, however, the weight and fat loss will begin to slow down as your body begins to adapt to the new routine.

1. *Calories.* Oftentimes, when you start a weight loss plan, you are tempted to dramatically lower your calorie intake. Severely restricting your calories can lead to weight loss trouble. When the body senses too large a decrease in calorie intake, it slows its metabolic rate to compensate (Homeostasis). While at first there will be weight loss as the body adjusts, once the body can regulate itself, you will require fewer calories to function. This creates hunger and prevents weight and fat loss. In addition, since you now need fewer calories, you will likely tire easier and your body will find ways for you to move less. To prevent this cycle, do not drastically cut calories. If you keep calorie intake slightly below your initial maintenance, your metabolism and energy levels can remain high during physical activities. Moreover, you body will not adapt to an extremely low calorie intake. *Tip: Only reduce your calorie intake by 10-15% maximum.*

2. *Supplementation.* Oftentimes when we decrease our caloric intake, we end up missing out on vital nutrients. At 1800 calories, you will barely be able to get all the nutrients from food, and if you are consuming below 1600 calories, it is highly unlikely that you will consume all of the necessary daily nutrients from food alone. Moreover, when you are deficient in vitamins and minerals, you body will break down your muscle to get the necessary nutrients. As a result, you lose muscle, which burns fat, and your metabolism will slow down. To combat this cycle, it is important to supplement your diet. Taking a daily *Multivitamin* along with an *Antioxidant* will help.

3. **Create a plan in stages for long term success.**
   Your body has an Internal Mechanism called a "Set Point" - similar to the temperature on a Thermostat. Your Genetics, Gender and the Choices you make determine what that set point is. Most initial results happen because the body is above your "Set Point". Imagine setting your home's thermostat to 80 Degrees. If the temperature is at 85, the air conditioning will switch on. However, once the room reaches 80, the cooling will stop. Your body works in a similar fashion.

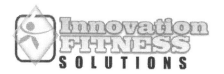
Weight Loss Stages:
I strongly recommend the use of a *Staged Weight Loss Plan.* I bring this up right now because you are about to be at the end of your First Stage. For the Non-Gym Fitness Event I recommend participating in Yoga or running a 5K or playing Golf. Something new that is a learned skill and challenging to the body, the soul and the mind.

Duration	3 Months	1 Month	2 Months	1 Month	2 Months	1 Month
Stage	Weight Loss	Weight Maintenance	Weight Loss	Weight Maintenance	Muscle Gain	Weight Maintenance
Focus	R.P.M.	Healthier Eating	R.P.M.	Non- Gym Fitness Event	Boost Metabolism	Finances, Relationships

**Revisit and Refocus your Life Quadrant on pages 34-35.

How to Get Past a Weight Loss Plateau: Proven Plateau Busters

Avoiding a plateau is a significant undertaking. Using the Staged Weight Loss Plan like the one listed is incredibly helpful, but even with all of the preparation to avoid a plateau you will inevitably see your weight/fat loss slow or stop. So, in preparation for this occurrence here are lists of action steps you can take to minimize the effects of a plateaus and to reenergize your body and mind to restart your results process.

Plateau Buster #1: Start Monitoring Body Fat, Not Just Scale Weight
Remember, it's not really about weight loss, but *fat loss*. The key to recognizing true fat loss plateaus is to carefully track both scale weight and body fat percentages.
Start measuring and tracking body at percentages, as well as weight, and monitor the change in muscle to body fat ratios, not just scale weight. Take your body fat percentage measurements once per month. Ask a Personal Trainer at your health club to perform the assessment. They most likely have the tools and experience to better assess your true body fat levels. As long as your body fat percentage is decreasing, you can be pretty sure that you haven't hit a weight loss plateau.

If you haven't lost any additional body fat in 2-3 weeks, then try one of the other weight loss plateau busters below.

Focused and Directed Action

Plateau Buster #2: Recalculate Your Calorie Requirements
As people lose weight or fat or gain muscle, their daily calorie needs changes as well. This is especially important if you've lost a significant amount of body fat or weight since the last time you did this calculation. As your weight decreases, so can your daily calorie requirements.
This could mean that you're eating more food than you need for your new weight. This can lead to your fat and weight loss progress stalling.
It's a good idea to recalculate your calorie requirements at least once every two months (use both formulas provided in this book). Use this new number to adjust your daily calorie intake based on your goals. If you continue to experience a plateau, keep reading.

Plateau Buster #3 Get Specific with Your Diet
Whenever someone says they've hit a "weight loss plateau", one of the first things I suggest is to take a very close look at diet and portions.
We're a Super-Size-Me nation and it's hard for even the most disciplined person to get a true sense of portions — and more importantly — to sustain this over the long haul. You may think your diet and portions are the same as two months ago when you were shedding body fat like crazy, but is this really the case now? If your sense of servings has gradually increased, the extra calories will add up and that can mean you will lose body fat more slowly. Go back to using a food scale for a few days a week and recheck your internal portion controls.

So get really meticulous about your diet for a few weeks. Here's how you do that:
Sign up for an on-line, calorie and exercise tracking websites like
www.dotfit.com/InnovationFitnessSolutions or www.Livestrong.com
Adjust your portions and eating habits based on what you are learning from your food log.
I recommend using the logging site and the food scale for at least one full week of each month.
There is no cure like an ounce of prevention!

Plateau Buster #4: Check Your Workout Routine and Activity Levels
Just like your diet, your exercise and activity habits can degrade as well. Intensity can drop, you get pressed for time and start cutting your workouts short; it gets cold outside and you become a little less active. Over time, these reductions in activity can start to chip away at how many calories you are actually burning each day.
Even a reduction of 50-100 extra calories burned from activity can have long term fat-loss and weight loss consequences. Over a period of 30 days, ending the day up 50 calories from working out with less duration or intensity can result in a gain of a half-pound of fat in a month.
The trick here is to use the same approach to your exercise and activity that we discussed earlier around diet. Track your activity and exercise by:
If you are not already, begin to journal your weight and resistance training exercise, as well cardio, using either the on-line option or trusty old pen and paper.

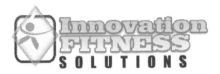

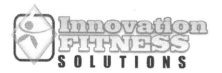

Check to see if you are still coming in at or around your goal targets for fat/weight loss. Use the same method of tracking activity at least one week per month. Continue to alter your workouts weekly and do not let your mind get stale with your workouts. A good rule of thumb is if you have memorized your weekly workouts and workout schedule so did your body (a long time ago…). Keep things fresh and your body will continue to respond for longer.

Plateau Buster # 5: Increase your total # of meals
People who eat smaller, more frequent meals every 2-3 hours have less propensity to over-eat, and they typically use their calories more efficiently as energy and for muscle recovery, versus storing the excess as body fat. Consider spreading your meals out over the day to see if it helps shock your system out of a plateau.
Tip: If you currently eat 3 meals then move to 4. If you are eating 4 meals then attempt 5 meals.

Plateau Buster # 6: Cycle Your Calories.
Calorie-cycling is a method of eating that alternates higher-calorie days with lower-calorie days in order prevent weight loss plateaus from developing in the first place.
IMPORTANT: I do not suggest this method for individual with bad craving or hunger problems. Gain control of those two issues first before you begin this method.

Calorie-cycling works because *on average across the week* you'll come in at an energy deficit that is adequate to produce the fat-loss you are looking for. For example, if you need to create a weekly calorie deficit of 3500 calories to lose one pound of fat a week, you'll spread that out unequally across seven days.
Let's say you are on a 2000 calorie diet (this is how many calories you need to eat to maintain your current weight).

Here's what your calories might look like day-to-day on a calorie cycle:

This accomplishes a larger calorie deficit average/week without starving yourself and feeds your body often enough as not to cause muscle loss.

Calorie Cycling:	
Monday:	1800 calories
Tuesday:	1600 calories
Wednesday:	2000 calories
Thursday:	1500 calories
Friday:	1700 calories
Saturday:	1600 calories
Sunday:	2000 calories

Transform Your Thinking.
Transform Your Body.
Transform Your Life.

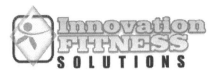

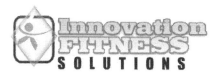

Good, Better, Best

Food choices for Plateau Busting

While general, occasional changes are good enough to make dramatic changes during the first 30-45 days of your transformation this simply does not hold true for the long term. Moving forward you are going to need to spend a bit more time making deliberate choices more times than not. Weight loss slows down and often stops cold for a while. Deliberately choosing more complex, more nutrient packed, low calories foods more often will improve your progress and your result.

Here are two lists of Best, Better and Bad food choices. Try to use the 4-4-2 rule. If you are choosing the best 4 out of 10, the Better 4 out of 10 and the Bad only 2 out of 10 then those cumulative choices will yield great long term gains for improving your health and keeping your calories down.

Technical Talk: This is called the Thermic Effect of Food

If your goal is to break down body fat, increase metabolism and feel your best now and in the future, it's important to understand how the quality of your food choices impact your results. The most important step in keeping energy level even throughout the day and maximize your metabolism is to eat a meal balanced in protein, carbohydrates and fat every three to four hours. This is the basis of a solid nutrition plan and staves off hunger which can lead to overeating and poor food choices.

The next step is to choose protein, carbohydrates and fats that are higher up on the quality of food chart. High quality foods are less processed, more natural and take longer to break down in your system (which causes your body to burn more calories.

Environmental control strategies:

1) Do not keep food on your counters.
2) Hide the junk. Show off the goods.
3) Leave the Griller on the counter. You'll use it more often.
4) Create a blockade to the sweets and chips.
5) Hang motivating pictures on your refrigerator.

1. Don't tempt yourself by keeping trigger foods around the house.
2. Pre Eat! Don't go to a party starving.
3. When you attend celebrations, don't station yourself near the buffet table.
4. When you shop, eat before you leave home.
5. You have got to add in life's little pleasures to succeed long term. Just set limits.

*See the complete list in the Support Material Section.

HIGHEST QUALITY FOODS

PROTEINS	CARBOHYDRATES	FATS

PROTEINS
- Beef
- Chicken
- Eggs
- Fish
- Turkey
- Soy Beans

CARBOHYDRATES
- Beans (fresh)
- Brown Rice
- Fruit
- Hot Cereals
- Vegetables
- Yams/Sweet Potatoes

FATS
- Avocado
- Flax Seed Oil
- Nuts (dry roasted or raw)
- Natural Nut Butters

MEDIUM QUALITY FOODS (these items are processed to some degree)

PROTEINS
- Cottage Cheese/ Yogurt
- Deli Meat
- Canned Meat
- Garden Burgers

CARBOHYDRATES
- Bread
- Beans - canned
- Cold Cereals
- Crackers/ Pretzels
- Pasta
- Potatoes

FATS
- Canola Oil
- Olives - canned
- Processed Nut Butters

LOW QUALITY FOODS (these items are the most processed)

PROTEINS
- Protein Powder
- Protein Bars

CARBOHYDRATES
- Chips
- White Rice
- Rice Cakes

FATS
- Mayonnaise
- Margarine
- Salad Dressings
- Sour Cream

What will you eat for dinner this evening?
Protein:
Carbohydrate:
Fat:
Calories:
Breakfast tomorrow?
Protein:
Carbohydrate:
Fat:
Calories:

Plan Ahead

71

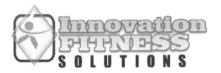

*The next chart is about calories: Focus on "Calorically Cheap and Healthy" foods for better long term results.

Calorically Expensive and Un-Healthy Foods to Avoid

- Baked goods such as cookies, crackers, cakes, etc.
- Margarine or partially hydrogenated oils
- Chinese food – most of the time
- Fried/sautéed foods
- 90% or below Ground Meat or when ordered out
- Cream soups/sauces (white or pink)
- Sauce – Puttinesca, Marsala, Picata
- Egg Yolks
- Cheeses – (The harder the cheese the higher the fat)
- Pastry products/cakes
- Most Deli Meats - Salami, bologna, pepperoni, etc
- Tuna or egg salad – store bought (any mayo based salads/sides)

Calorically Expensive Foods That Are Healthy

- Nuts (all types), Olive Oil, Avocados
- 2% cottage cheese
- Salmon (omega 3's)
- Dried Fruit

Calorically Cheap Foods That Are Healthy

- Lite breads (whole/Multi grain, High Fiber, High Pro)
- Sweet Potatoes/Yams, Brown Rice, Oatmeal/ Oat Bread
- Whole Wheat pasta
- Sauces – Marinara, Fra Diavlo, Tomato
- Chicken (skinless breast)
- Low fat/salt ham, Turkey (fresh roast)
- Low fat cheeses (cottage)
- Eye round roast beef, Buffalo (ground or steak), Ostrich
- Pork tenderloin and center-cut boneless chops
- Cod, Pollack, Haddock, Orange Ruffy, Tilapia

Appetite Control:

1) *Know what foods trigger your appetite* and do not purchase them or keep them in your home.
2) *Eat slowly.* Use a 1-10 scale and determine how quickly you complete your meal. Aim to slow down to a 5 or 6 speed of eating.
3) *Listen to your bodies hunger.* Use that same 1-10 scale. Determine your actual hunger and fill your plate accordingly. Most of us what eat all that we serve ourselves even if we are not hungry for it.
4) *Eat more Fiber.* Eating high fiber foods increase your feeling of fullness.
5) *Brush your teeth* immediately following your meal or chew a piece of sugar free gum to end your eating session.

*Think Win-Win
There is no BAD,
Only Better*

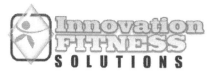

Days 61 – 90 Articles - Forms of Self Defeating Thoughts

All too often it is the stuff between your ears that prevents you from true, lasting changes and transformation. We become our own worst enemy and usually make too much of our setbacks while not giving ourselves enough credit for our successes. The people that succeed the most tend to be their own cheerleaders! Avoid these mental scenarios and you will live a happier, more fulfilled life AND transform your body! We suggest "Flipping it" by creating a list of steps you will do.

Example: *I know that I usually go full force into a diet and exercise program. When I get discouraged by eating a dessert or missing a workout I can't seem to get remotivated.*
Solution: *I know that that strategy has not worked in the past, so now I will make allowances for changes to plans and as long as I keep moving forward with progress I will not give up!*

---

1. All or nothing - thinking Many of us tend to think in black-and white categories. If a situation falls short of perfect, we see it as a total failure. No one thing will make you gain or lose weight. You will be successful because of repeated efforts over time.

2. Mental filter If you pick out a single negative detail and dwell on it exclusively, so that your vision of all of reality becomes darkened, like the drop of ink that discolors a beaker of water. Example: You receive many positive comments about your progress and weight loss/appearance, but one of them says something mildly critical or you are not at the final scale/# goal you obsess about this reaction for days and ignore all the positive feedback. Discounting the positive takes the joy out of life and makes you feel inadequate and unrewarded.

4. Magnification You exaggerate the importance of your setbacks, problems and shortcomings, or you minimize the importance of your desirable qualities.

5. Emotional reasoning and Should v Will You assume that your negative emotions necessarily reflect the way things really are: 'I am not doing well in changing my appearance/life. Or 'I feel guilty for eating that "bad food". I must be a rotten person.' Or I feel so inferior. This means I'm a second-rate person.' Or 'I feel hopeless. I must really be hopeless.' These types of statements set you up for eventual failure because there will be a time when you will not be perfect. Asking 'Will' questions is much more helpful, Realistic and Maintainable. What am I willing to do now and forever? What will I be able to live with and keep doing? These types of strategic questions will help to create long term success.

6. Labeling - Labeling is an extreme form of all-or-nothing thinking. Instead of saying "I made a mistake." you attach a negative label to yourself: "I'm a loser." Labeling is quite irrational because you are not the same as what you do. Human beings exist. but 'fools,' 'losers,' and 'jerks' do not. These labels are useless abstractions that lead to anger, anxiety, frustration, and low self- esteem. Labeling something as "Good" or "Bad" is not a complete story. Putting everything and its' effects into context (Big Picture) is an essential component to reaching a large, long term goal.

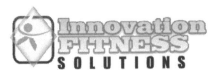

Getting over Failures and moving forward.

- ✦ What is past is all said and done. What remains to be seen is what I can bring to my present and future.
- ✦ Better for me to concentrate on what I'm doing today rather than on what I did or didn't do before. What I do today will shape my tomorrows.
- ✦ The past isn't going to get any better!
- ✦ Poor decisions made in the past do not have to be repeated in the present.
- ✦ Because something once happened doesn't mean that it has to continue to happen.
- ✦ No matter how bad any event was, I do not have to allow it to continue to have a negative influence on my life. I cannot rewrite history and change what has already happened.
- ✦ I'm going to put more money down on what can yet be made to happen than on what has already happened.
- ✦ Feeling sorry for myself, angry toward others, guilty, or ashamed for getting the short end of the stick in the past will only continue to keep me from achieving happiness in the present and future.
- ✦ What I tell myself today is much more important than what others have told me in the past.

Reality Check

There is a vast amount of confusing information available regarding Dieting and Exercise Magic. It is important to know the difference between Reality and Myth. Here are a few of the most popular and potentially damaging Myths and the concrete concepts in which to rely.

Myth #1: You Can Target One Area of Your Body for Weight Loss. AKA: Spot Reduction
Reality: The muscle does not "OWN" the fat that surrounds it.
This is a myth, pure and simple. No matter how much exercise you do for a specific region of the body, it's physically impossible to lose body fat in a targeted area. Worse yet, the areas of your body that gain fat the fastest are the last to see it go. Fat is gained or lost throughout the entire the body. But don't despair. Just because you are not losing fat from exactly where you want to does not mean you will not lose it from there eventually. It will just take a bit longer. Stay consistent.

Myth #2: If your goal is body fat reduction, you'll burn more fat in your target heart rate zone; if you go over it you will burn muscle
Reality: If you're maintaining a calorie deficit, then the harder you work the more calories you'll burn and the faster you'll lose fat

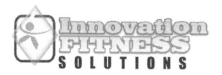

Myth #3: You Do Not Have To Count Calories
Reality: Counting Calories Is Important
You definitely need to count calories in order to lose weight. People tend to overestimate their physical activity and underestimate their calories. As a matter of fact multiple studies conclude that the higher an individual's BMI is, the more they tend to miscalculate. Do not rely on eyeballing your caloric intake or trying to estimate it. Instead, be sure to journal every day for Food and Fitness Activities. To make it easier for you to quantify your physical activity, wear a pedometer. Do this every day. Consistency is important for dieting. Sure, this is not easy. But if you want to lose weight, this is important to do on a daily basis.

Myth #4: Eat Three Times a Day and Do Not Snack
Reality: Eat consistently throughout the day and maintain your Calorie Intake
Remember, it is all about calories. You can eat three times a day or six times a day, as long as you do not exceed your daily caloric intake. However, you should have at least three meals a day to structure your daily eating, so you do not become too hungry. And if you eat six times a day, the meals will be smaller ones.

Myth #5: Lifting Weights Can Make You Look Bulky.
Reality: This is a myth that deters many women from strength training. In fact, what determines the amount of muscle bulk a person has is largely dependent on genetic factors. So for the typical woman, and the typical man, the chances of looking like Arnold Schwarzenegger are very slim.
Weight training is also an important part of any exercise plan, according to the American Heart Association web site. While aerobic activities help your heart and lungs and stretching improves your flexibility, weight training will improve your strength and endurance, and a combination of all three makes for an optimal exercise plan. Weight training also burns significant calories over many other forms of exercise.

Myth #6: Carbohydrates Make You Fat
Reality: Carbohydrates Are Necessary For a Balanced Diet.
Carbohydrates do not make you fat; extra calories do. Whether you eat them in the form of carbohydrates, fats, or protein, carbohydrates are the preferred source of energy for the body. If you do not eat enough carbohydrates, the body will eventually break down other tissues, primarily muscle, for energy. This, in turn, will slow your metabolism and your fat burning capacity down making it harder to lose weight. What you want to do is eat carbohydrates in moderation and select carbohydrate sources from fruits, vegetables, and whole grains.

"You don't plan to fail, you fail to plan!"

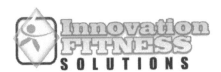
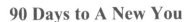
Myth #7: Avoid Fats
Reality: **Fats Increase Your Sense of Fullness**
Fat has more calories per gram than protein and carbohydrate so cutting back on fat will help you to reduce calories. However, you do not want to avoid fat completely. Studies show that fat contributes to a sense of satiety and adds flavor to many foods. Eliminating fat from your diet will increase your hunger. Avoid saturated and trans fats found in meat, poultry skin, high-fat dairy, eggs, processed baked goods and fried foods. Instead, choose monounsaturated and polyunsaturated fats found in fish, nuts and vegetable oils (e.g., olive oil, canola oil, peanut oil).

Myth #8: Do Not Worry About Dieting — Just Exercise
Reality: **Exercising Alone Is Not Enough**
You probably will not be able to work out enough to make up for eating a huge meal. Exercise alone does not keep you in a calorie deficit required to lose weight. For example, if you eat a slice of apple pie a la mode that is 500 calories, you will have to walk briskly for two hours to burn off those calories. Bottom line, you will not lose weight unless you also cut calories.

> If you Caloric Maintenance is 1500 calories you could eat at any time you want as long as you do not go in excess of that #. However, if you have a #1 Supersized Meal form a Fast Food Establishment and a $5.00 Coffee that will cost you about 2000 calories. If you ate this by 2pm you have already gone over the allotment for the day.
> Time is irrelevant. Calories in v Calories Out hold the truth.

Myth #9: Never Eat After 8 PM
Fact: **Calories Do Not Own Watches**
What is important is how many calories you consume throughout the day; not when you eat them. Many people intentionally save 200 to 300 calories to eat at night. Sure, eating a big meal before you go to bed may give you some indigestion, but it will not necessarily result in weight gain. Eating at night may be the best time for you. You are at home, the kids are in bed, and you have time to enjoy your food. Bottom line, it is possible to have a late snack or meal and stick to your diet plan.

Myth #10: If You Eat Well, You Do Not Need to Supplement Your Diet with a Multivitamin
Reality: **Nobody Eats Perfectly 365 Days Of The Year**
Regardless of whether you eat well or not, it is very difficult to consume all of the necessary vitamins and minerals on a daily basis, especially if you are following a low calorie diet. Consuming the recommended amounts of all vitamins and minerals allows you to maximize exercise performance, body fat reduction, lean tissue development and your health. If your body is deficient in inadequacies, any nutrient, the body will break down muscle tissue to release more nutrients. As a result, your metabolism may slow down slightly due to a reduction in muscle mass. Supplementing with a daily multivitamin also allows you to compensate for any nutritional inadequacies.

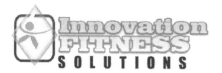

Myth #11: You Cannot Have Alcohol If You are On a Diet
Reality: **Alcohol Has Calories, But When Consumed in Moderation Can Fit Into Your Meal Plan**

Liquid calories from alcohol can really contribute to weight gain. When you drink alcoholic beverages, you do not tend to compensate by eating less because most beverages only satisfy thirst and do not contribute to a feeling full. If you drink alcohol, do so in moderation, and choose lighter drink options such as a 12-ounce light beer (110 calories), a 6-ounce wine spritzer (60 calories), 5 ounces of wine (120-130 calories), or try alternating alcoholic drinks with non-alcoholic drinks.

Myth #12: Doing cardio first thing in the morning on an empty stomach is the best way to lose fat. What do you think?
Reality: Well, it is a way, but not necessarily the best way. When you awaken, your body is in a fasting metabolic state and burning fewer calories per unit of time than usual. Consuming some food will perk your metabolic rate up (hence, the term "breakfast" – breaking the fast). Additionally, glycogen stores are depleted by as much as 80%. This will adversely affect your ability to work out at a high intensity and may cause weakness and dizziness and lead to early fatigue. If meal preparation time is an issue, the use of a meal replacement drink can be helpful.

Rebounding from Mental Roadblocks:

1. Think Inclusion not Restriction. Don't pass up favorite foods or deprive yourself completely. Moderate consumption is the key. Don't let perfect get in the way of good!

2. If you fall off the wagon do not think that all is lost. It's not. If you overdo it just go back to your regular plan the next day and move a little more.

3. Have FUN! You are doing something good for yourself!

Don't let perfect get in the way of good!

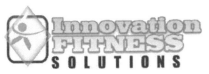

Realistic, Progressive and Maintainable Tips: Food

Dieting is hard so we recommend that you do not do it!
Trimming a little bit of calories here and there can do wonders for your weight and health. It is not always about eating less; sometimes it is about eating smarter. Skimming off calories is easier than you think. Challenge yourself to implement one new strategy everyday for eating and one for exercise

All it takes are a few small efforts to help trim excess calories. **Pick two strategies a day** and you will cut 100 calories, burn 100 more calories a day (a 15- to 20-minute walk will do the trick) and you will lose almost half a pound a week. That may not sound like much, but it adds up to 20 pounds a year! The more tricks you incorporate the more pounds you will lose. Little things yield huge rewards.

1. Leave the cheese off your sandwich. Have your sandwich without the cheese and you can use the cheese as part of a snack. *Caloric Saving: 100*

2. Use 1 cup skim milk instead of 1 cup whole milk. *Caloric Saving: 70*

3. Use a nonstick spray instead of oil. If you need liquid, use a low sodium and low fat chicken or vegetable broth. Make every meal in a nonstick pan, and you will automatically save at least **100 calories** every time by eliminating the butter, margarine or oil used to grease the pan. When sautéing or frying, simply coat nonstick pans with a spritz of vegetable oil cooking spray (0 calories). Every tablespoon of oil or butter that you do not use. *Caloric Saving: 125*

4. Sip on flavored seltzer or diet soda instead of regular soda. For every 12 ounce can of soda you substitute with seltzer or diet soda you will have saved some major calories. *Caloric Saving: 160*

5. Use 1 tablespoon of light mayonnaise instead of 1 tablespoon regular mayonnaise. *Caloric Saving: 75*

6. Eat 2 tablespoons less ice cream. You will not even miss it. *Caloric Saving: 70*

7. Drink 4 ounces less juice. Or better yet, skip the juice all together and eat the whole fruit instead and be more satisfied. *Caloric Saving: 110*

8. Use 1 tablespoon less cream cheese. Most breakfast sandwiches have more than is necessary. Each tablespoon of cream cheese has 50 calories and 5 grams of fat. Light cream cheese has only 35 calories and 2.5 grams of fat with all the taste and flavor. *Caloric Saving: 50+*

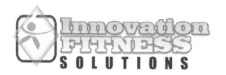

9. Order small fries instead of large fries. An order of small fries from your typical fast food restaurant has 225 calories and 11 grams of fat and a large order of fries has 500 and 25 grams of fat. *Caloric Saving: 275*

10. When making burgers, meatballs or meatloaves, substitute 4 ounces ground extra-lean or lean turkey for 4 ounces ground beef. *Caloric Saving: Up to 265 Calories per 4 oz of meat*

11. Make weekly shopping a habit by setting a specific day and time when you can always go. Without healthy foods on hand, you may be tempted to improvise by hitting fast-food and convenience stores, where nearly everything is high-fat and high-calorie. *Caloric Saving: The Sky's the Limit*

12. Satisfy your cravings with a low-calorie treat, about 150 calories. Limit rich desserts (most have about 500 calories) to when you go out for a nice dinner, no more than once a week. *Caloric Saving:350 Calories a day for six days, or 2,100 Calories/WK*

13. Incorporate protein into your breakfast. Research has shown that the more you eat earlier on in the day, the less you eat as the day goes on. Remember dairy has protein in it so cereal with some low-fat or fat-free milk may just do the trick to keep you feeling satisfied. *Caloric Savings: 200[+]*

14. Choose whole fruit. They are full of fiber and water, so your stomach will fill up sooner, causing you to eat less with fewer calories. Studies show, that people who eat at least three apples or pears a day lose weight. Try substituting that mid-afternoon vending machine meal. *Caloric Savings: 220*

15. Blot that pizza. Pat your slice with a napkin to cut anywhere from a teaspoon to a tablespoon of unnecessary grease -- and calories. *Caloric Saving: 50-140*

16. Be a kid again. You do not to totally abandon that fast food lunch, we understand, *sometimes* it may be unavoidable. It can fit into your meal plan if you order smaller sizes. Instead of that Quarter Pounder with Cheese and large fries, opt for the Hamburger Happy Meal. *Caloric Savings: 490*

17. Craving chocolate? Trade in that chocolate candy bar for a sugar-free, reduced-calorie Jell-O chocolate pudding snack with a tablespoon of nonfat whipped cream topping. *Caloric Saving: 185*

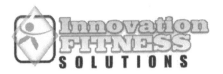

18. What about a Barbecue? Have that hot dog, but bulk it up. Load that dog with some pickles, onions and sauerkraut -- these condiments are fiber-rich and will fill you up and keep you going back for seconds… or thirds. *Caloric Saving: 250*

19. Think before you drink. Choose light beer or wine instead of one of those sugar-saturated frozen drinks: A bottle of light beer has 100 calories and a 4-oz glass of wine has 80 calories, while a strawberry daiquiri has about 300 and a margarita 340. *Caloric Saving: 200-260*

20. I scream, you scream, we all scream for ice cream. But we do not want all those calories. Spoil yourself with chocolate sorbet instead of chocolate ice cream. *Caloric Saving: 125*

RESTAURANT STRATEGIES

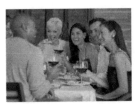

➧ Be assertive. Do not be shy. Ask the waiter if a dish can be slightly adjusted. Restaurants rely on customer satisfaction and will go to great lengths to ensure that you get what you want. This can also be done with the sides. Sides from one entrée can often be substituted with sides from a different entrée. If it comes with mashed potatoes, ask for a side of veggies instead.

➧ Ask for double vegetables instead of rice or mashed potatoes. Make sure the veggies are steamed.

➧ Order from the "healthy, lite or low fat" entrées on the menu. Most chains will even list the calories and nutritional content of such foods. Check the on-line menu before visiting the restaurant.

➧ If you are a member of the "Clean your plate club" You could ask the server to wrap up half the entrée before they bring it out. "Pre Doggie bag."

➧ Check the menu before you leave home. Today most restaurants especially chain restaurants have websites with their menu options. If there is nothing you feel that can be easily altered, you can decide to go to a different restaurant.

Consistency:
Just because you had a "good week" doesn't mean you should give yourself the license to eat everything that passes by on the weekends. Factor the little extras into your daily intake.
It ALL counts.

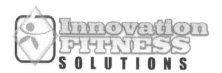

Better Bad Food Choices – Fast Food

Fast-food is known for being high in calories, fat and sodium. However, most fast-food restaurants have now added healthier options to their menus. To make better food choices and save additional calories, follow some of these simple guidelines:

- Try to limit fast-food to once or twice per week.
- Avoid sauces like special sauce, mayonnaise, sour cream, butter, cheese sauces, gravy and tartar sauce.
- Avoid super-sizing your meal.
- Choose fat-free or low-fat milk, diet soda, unsweetened iced tea, or water instead of regular sodas and milkshakes.
- Order the smallest size burger (e.g., a single hamburger instead of a double hamburger) and leave off the cheese.
- Select grilled/broiled chicken and fish sandwiches (and salads) instead of fried/ breaded chicken and fish sandwiches (and salads).
- Choose a side salad (with low-fat or fat-free dressing on the side) or plain baked potato (with salsa and vegetables) instead of fries and onion rings.
- Select a thin crust pizza with vegetable toppings instead of a deep dish pizza with meat toppings like sausage and pepperoni.
- Avoid the loaded baked potato (with cheese, sour cream, butter) – instead add extra salsa or vegetables.
- Choose fruit and/or yogurt for dessert.
- Note that plain bagels and English muffins are less damaging than croissants and pastries.
- Choose wraps or sandwiches on whole wheat bread or pita when possible.
- Choose baked chips instead of regular chips.
- Review the nutritional facts for your favorite fast-food restaurant meals either online or at the restaurant before making your food selections.

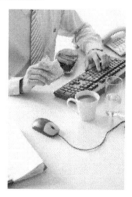

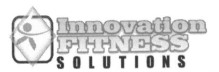
Key Points: Days 61-90

✓ Eat a balanced breakfast when you wake up.
✓ Do not go more than 3 to 4 hours without eating (unless you are sleeping).
✓ Try to eat 3 meals and 1-2 snacks per day.
✓ Eat a snack composed of carbohydrates, protein, and fat within 45 minutes after completing a workout to help repair damaged muscle and replenish muscle glycogen (energy) stores.
✓ Keep healthy snacks with you.
✓ Always eat with a plan.
✓ Persistence, Commitment, Belief and Environmental Control
✓ Schedule your workouts and movement.
✓ Plan to do something every day that will bring you closer to your goal.
✓ Mentally prepare yourself for setbacks. Be resilient in adversity and determined to find a solution.
✓ Take your Multi Vitamin daily.
✓ Stay Positive and Find a reason to smile often.
✓ New strategies and habits = A NEW YOU.
✓ Don't give up! Don't EVER give up!

Weekly Report Card: Days 61-90

Rate your progress on a 1(Low) – 5(Great) scale.

Food

Did you keep your Food Journal?	Avg # of meals daily?
Are you planning ahead: ☐	Meal Timing?
Avg. H2O Daily: ☐	Quality of food:
Sleeping Well: ☐ Hours:	Energy Level:
Meal Timing: (Hours):	Speed of Eating:
Coffee/ Caloric Drinks:	Alcohol:
Multi Vitamin:	

Fitness

Accidental Exercise (Daily):	Cardio sessions (Week):
Exercise Intensity?	Strength Training Sessions:

Mental Fitness

	Success:
Motivation Level:	Weight Loss:
Did you read?	Inches Lost:

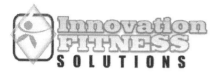

Support Material

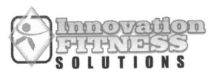

Quick Reference Guide:

Your Formula for Daily Success:

Read this daily for continued **inspiration**.

- ✓ Accept No Limits
- ✓ Conquer Doubt
- ✓ Put Off Procrastination
- ✓ Don't Quit
- ✓ Live In the Solution
- ✓ Take Responsibility
- ✓ See Yourself Succeed
- ✓ Focus On Ideas
- ✓ Every Circumstance Has Two Sides
- ✓ Master Your Fears
- ✓ Persist
- ✓ Directed Thoughts
- ✓ Be Blind To Failure
- ✓ Decide To Grow
- ✓ Create Your Own Circumstance
- ✓ Problems Bring Lessons
- ✓ Persistence
- ✓ Identify Your Vision
- ✓ Thoughts Create your Behavior
- ✓ Control Your Destiny
- ✓ Expect to lose weight over time
- ✓ Modify your Food and Fitness plan as you lose weight
- ✓ Focus on both Long Term and Short Term Goals
- ✓ Find out how many calories are in your favorite foods
- ✓ Commit to losing weight
- ✓ Strive for consistency
- ✓ Your habits determine your outcome
- ✓ Make small changes to see big results
- ✓ Be prepared for roadblocks

Your List of Daily Questions:

Read this daily for continued **direction**.

- Did I Eat Breakfast?
- Did I Take My Multi Vitamin?
- Did I Read for 10 minutes today?
- Did I Journal Today?
- Did I Find Ways to Add In 'Surprise exercise' Today?
- Did I Stay Positive Today?
- Did I find 10 Minutes to Be with My Thoughts?
- How Have I Helped Myself Today?
- Did I eat balanced meals today (P,C,F)?
- Did I eat every 3-4 hours, not going more than 5 hours without eating?
- How many calories did I consume today?
- How many calories did I burn today?
- List out the 'Surprise Exercise' that I performed today.
- How much time did I spend reading today?
- What were my reasons to smile today?

What is the most important thing I can do today to keep me on track?

***Print out at

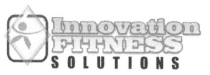

Stuff You Should Know – Frequently Asked Questions

Food

1. **How do you determine an appropriate calorie level for me?**
   - Each individual requires a different amount of calories and movement to attain their goal. Use two separate scientific formulas (Harris – Benedict Equation and Katch – McCardle) to most accurately estimate your caloric intake.
   - There are multiple factors that are accounted for when figuring out how much you should eat including age, gender, bodyweight, lean body mass, body fat, activity level, genetics, and diet history. Estimating caloric intake is not an exact science but with the formulas and monitoring and journaling you can figure out what will work for you.
   - Your caloric needs change daily with the changes in hunger, appetite and movement so consistently monitoring the above factors will help to save you time and energy in attaining your goal.

2. **What is the correct percentage of protein, fat, and carbohydrate that I should be consuming?**
   - There isn't a "perfect" ratio for everyone. This, like your caloric requirements are different for each individual. More important are the recommendations or ranges set forth by The American Dietetic Association. The recommendations for each of the macronutrients of total calorie intake are as follows: Where you end up in the range based on your caloric needs, appetite and type of movement.
     - Carbohydrates: 45-65%
     - Protein: 15-25%
     - Fat: 10-30%

3. **Why do I need to drink 8-10 glasses of water per day?**
   - According to the American Dietetic Association, the human body is made up of 50 to 75 percent water. Therefore, replenishing your body's water supply is crucial for proper function. Recently studies have illustrated that foods with high water content will contribute to your daily water consumption.
   - There is a lot of confusion surrounding water intake. There have been reports stating that it, *flushes fat, fills you up, and increases your metabolism.* There is some truth in all of these reports. Nevertheless, alone, water will not make one lose weight.
   - On the other hand, if you are drinking caloric beverages and begin to substitute these beverages with water you will be eliminating some extra and unnecessary calories which will in turn, contribute to weight loss. Still, with or without the myths, there is no disputing that water is good for us and is the superior choice among other beverages.

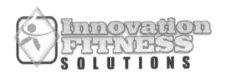

4. Do I have to count calories?

- No. However, you must become more aware or conscious of where your calories are coming from. It is important to know how much you are eating and how much you are moving to accurately understand and predict what the outcome is going to be. Without this knowledge you rely on guesswork which most often is not a long-term solution

- The only way the body can get smaller is if the total energy intake is less than the total energy expended.

5. Do I need to follow a strict diet or cook meals?

- There are three ways that you can be successful
  1) Follow the menu plans exactly.
  2) Follow the menu plans and utilize the appropriate exchanges.
  3) Add freedom and flexibility, using the menu plan as a guide.

- There is no best way to do this. The method that you choose will depend on the goals that you choose and your personality type. If you are an individual that does best following a "strict " protocol then option creating a menu template will work best for you.

- Whichever method you choose, as long as you are accountable for your actions and aware of your movement and food choices, you should be successful long-term.

- Cooking your own meals would be incredibly helpful not only for your weight loss goals but also to help improve your health. The more control you have over your surroundings the better your awareness of what you're doing. Increasing your awareness of your food intake will increase the likelihood that you will be successful.

- With that said, you can still attain your fitness goals relying on fast food, restaurants and frozen, re-heated meals. Remember, you gain weight when you consume more than you burn off.

6. Do I have to eat even if I am not hungry?

- It is important to eat every 3-4 hours. By doing so you can keep your energy levels (blood sugar) stable and most importantly prevent hunger. When you go too long without eating a snack or meal you'll eventually get hungry. Most people will make impulsive food decisions when hungry and end up overeating. Be sure to never go longer than 5 hours between meals.

7. Am I allowed to drink alcohol?

- Think in terms of accountability for your actions not elimination of foods and/or drink.
- Be accountable for your foods and liquids. Burn more calories than you consume and fit the alcohol in.

Inclusion, Not Restriction

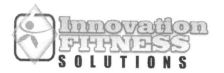

8. Do I have to keep a food journal?

- Food journaling is extremely important. Consider this: can you accurately recall every single thing that you ate and drank exactly one month ago? We didn't think so.
- The more frequently you track how much you move and how much you eat, the better decisions can be made regarding your solution. Ask yourself this: Is my goal short term or long term? If you answered long term then guesswork has no place in your solution.
- Journaling is necessary if you do not have a complete understanding of food amounts and need counseling on making better choices.
- There are multiple levels of compliance with food journaling. Some people track everything from foods eaten, calories, protein, carbohydrates, fats, and timing and some just jot down the foods eaten. I recommend journaling of some sort for the first 90 days to gain insight into your habits (good and bad).

9. I've tried many different diets, why will this one be any different?

- The known, inarguable rules to how people gain and lose weight have been established for years. Most weight loss methods focus on one aspect of Fitness/Weight Loss success, leaving you to fend for yourself on the other aspects. These attempts by the dieter are well meaning but incomplete.
- IFS is a complete coaching and education system. We will move you forward in all aspects of your fitness quest.

10. Do I have to eat special pre-packaged meals?

- No. I suggest as a strategy to plan ahead and prevent overeating that you stock your freezer with healthy, frozen meals like 'Healthy Choice' or 'Lean Cuisine' or 'Weight Watchers' meals.
- Incorporate these meals can be helpful as they are "controlled calorie meals" but they're no rules in your success. Whatever you can do and keep doing is what will work for you.

11. Do I have to give up my favorite foods?

- No. Have you ever attempted to cut out your favorite foods before? How did it work out for you? More than likely you lost a few pounds but eventually gained them back.
- The goal is to be aware of your habits and tweak them to work for you and allow you to control your outcome. There are no such things as fattening foods. Some are healthier than others but all foods have the potential to make you gain weight.

> Transform Your Thinking.
> Transform Your Body.
> Transform Your Life.

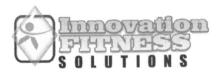

Fitness

1. **How much cardiovascular and weight/ resistance training should I be doing weekly?**
   - The answer to this question is completely dependent on your goal. Most athletes will need to do at least 4-5 days weekly of weight training and cardiovascular work plus sports specific practice and training.
   - For most novice fat loss clients it actually is much less. Two to three days weekly should be sufficient when you begin a Fat Loss plan.
   - Keep in mind that we are implementing strategies for Food Intake and Energy Expenditure. There is no need to rely on excessive cardio exercise.

2. **What's the best cardiovascular exercise to lose weight?**
   - The simple answer is anything that you will enjoy doing.
   - Many exercise participants create undue stress for themselves trying to find the "magic exercise" that burns the most calories in the shortest period of time. The reality is that this is only a short term solution. Your body is incredibly adaptive which requires you to change your workout (both Cardio and Resistance) on a regular basis.
   - I suggest starting with the exercise that you enjoy the most and manipulate the intensity for 3-4 weeks. At that point you will be ready to change your mode and force the body to start adjusting to something new. This will keep you burning the most calories in every workout.

3. **How many repetitions are best when weight training for weight loss?**
   - The goal of resistance training while in a fat loss plan is to burn the most calories in the least amount of time and to increase tonicity (muscle hardness/definition). The repetition range should be altered based on how long you have been doing the same type of program.
   - Remember: your body adapts to all new stimuli. The higher the frequency, the quicker the body adapts. It is important to make changes to your exercise type, repetition range; weight lifted and exercise order frequently.

4. **How many calories will I burn, on average, during a one-hour workout?**
   - Based on the research done by the National Institute on Health and the Taylor Code (an estimate of energy expenditure during exercise), you can burn between 300-600 calories per hour during resistance training and 200-500 calories per hour during cardio exercise.
   - If your goal is to increase calorie expenditure during exercise, it is essential that you keep your exercise program fresh and new. Making changes to your exercises, exercise order, sets, reps or amount of weight lifted will spark the body to burn more calories during and after the workout
   - There are multiple factors that will change this estimate:
     - Body Weight, Conditioning, Intensity of Movement

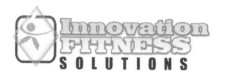
5. **When doing a workout that combines both cardio and weight resistance training, is it more beneficial to do weights first and then cardio or vice versa? Why?**
- Recent research from the nationally accredited personal training certifications recommend an exercise order as follows:
    1. Cardio Warm-up, Dynamic Warm-Up/ Stretching, Resistance Training, Flexibility, Cardio Exercise, Cool Down.
- However, if you are crunched for time and/or get bored doing resistance training prior to cardio, don't fret. Movement, no matter what order, will always be beneficial to calorie burning and improving health over not moving.
- For fat loss, the goal is to maintain tone and increase caloric burn during the workout. With that in mind, the exercise order is not nearly as important for an event athlete.
- For specific athletic events this will also change depending on the goal. An individual who is a strength athlete will be best suited to do a warm-up followed by resistance training than cardio. An athlete who is specific to endurance that utilizes resistance training for strength purposes will be better off focusing on their specific sport needs first.

6. **How should I measure my success?**
- There are multiple ways to measure success. The physical methods will be your bodyweight, your body fat percentage, how your clothes are fitting and your ability to perform your workout activities and activities of daily living better and more efficiently.
- The psychological measures will be how much better and more confident you are feeling about yourself. The improvements to your self esteem and your quality of life are endless when proper eating and exercise become a part of your life.
- I also strongly urge you to take 'Before and After' photos. Photos can be an extremely positive way to provide positive feedback. The day to day changes are incrementally small but when seen over the course of 1, 2 or more months, the visual aid can be staggering.

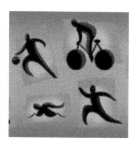

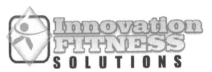

Nutrition for Weight Loss

BALANCING MEALS: PROTEIN, FATS, AND CARBOHYDRATES

Proteins, fats and carbohydrates, also known as macronutrients, all play a role in the growth and development and muscle and in the loss of fat. There are many diets out there that may recommend avoiding one of these macronutrients. However, it is the combination of proteins, fats and carbohydrates that enables your metabolism and your body to work properly.

PROTEIN
FACTS ABOUT PROTEIN:

1) The body uses proteins for a number of reasons. Protein is used to develop new cells, maintain tissues, and produce new proteins that make is possible to perform basic bodily functions. About half of dietary protein consumed goes into making enzymes. Enzymes are proteins that have specific tasks such as digesting food and making and dividing new cells. Every function that our body performs from seeing to thinking requires nerve cells to send signals back and forth to each other. These messages are transported via chemicals called neurotransmitters. Protein is required for manufacturing neurotransmitters, in addition to playing a critical role in the immune system and water balance.

2) All proteins are made up of building blocks called amino acids. There are 22 amino acids which are broken down into two categories, *essential* and *nonessential*. *Essential* amino acids must come from dietary sources because they cannot be made by the body. Whereas *nonessential* amino acids, are not required to be eaten as they can be made by the body.

3) The prevalent sources of protein in our diets are animal foods such as chicken, meat, fish, cheese, and eggs. However, plant proteins are believed to be healthier because of their lower fat content. Plant protein is found in beans, lentils, nuts, soy and seeds. However, every food, except for pure fats (oil and lard) or pure sugar, contain at least some protein.

SUGGESTIONS FOR ADDITION OF PROTEIN IN MEAL PLANNING

Protein should be included in every meal and snack. Combining protein at every meal will allow you to feel more satisfied. Protein is filling and takes longer to digest than carbohydrates alone, and will result in being able to get to the next meal or snack with ease without causing you to overeat. A simple rule to follow is, "no carbohydrate should be eaten alone and a protein needs to be included".

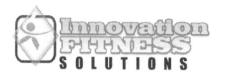

90 Days to A New You

Protein has the ability to stimulate the metabolism. Every time food is ingested, the body has to burn a certain number of calories just to digest the food eaten. This is often referred to as the thermic effect of food. Whenever protein is consumed, approximately 20% of the calories are used for digestion and assimilation of the food since protein is more difficult to digest than carbohydrates or fats. Protein has the greatest thermic effect on the metabolism; carbohydrate and fat have values of only 8% and 2%, respectively. Therefore, incorporating a moderate amount of protein at each meal or snack can help boost the metabolism.

FATS
FATS: THE GOOD, THE BAD, AND THE UGLY
Whenever you eat it is important to balance protein, carbohydrates and fat. This is especially important to remember as you try to change your body composition since each of these components are necessary for your body to function. Fats, however, can be tricky. Though we want to include fats since they provide the flavor and aroma to our food, we need to realize that not all fats are created equal. Understanding the different types of fats is especially important since the mix of fats in your diet may affect your cholesterol level and your heart.

TYPES OF FAT
There are four types of fats: monounsaturated, polyunsaturated, saturated and trans-fats. The first three listed occur naturally, whereas trans-fats are produced from a process known as hydrogenation. The following chart gives an overview of the types of fats and their effects on your cholesterol.

Type of Fat	Main Source	Effect on Cholesterol Levels
Monounsaturated	Olive oil, canola oil, peanut oil; olives; cashews, almonds, peanuts, and most other nuts; avocados	Lowers LDL (bad cholesterol) and Raises HDL (good cholesterol)
Polyunsaturated	Fish; corn, soybean, safflower, and sunflower oils	Lowers LDL and HDL
Saturated	Coconut, palm, and palm kernel oils; whole milk, butter, cheese, and ice cream; red meat; chocolate; coconuts and coconut milk	Raises LDL and HDL
Trans	Most commercial baked goods; most margarines; vegetable shortening; partially hydrogenated vegetable oil; many fast foods; deep-fried chips	Raises LDL and Lowers HDL

91

www.InnovationFitnessSolutions.com

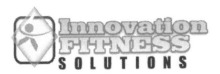
RECOMMENDATIONS FOR FAT INTAKE

The bottom line is that we need to replace the bad fats (saturated and trans-fats) with good fats (mono- and polyunsaturated fats). However, it is also important to note that all fat, regardless of good or bad, contains the same number of calories. Therefore, keep your fat intake to 20-30% of your total daily calorie intake.

CARBOHYDRATES
FACTS ABOUT CARBOHYDRATES

1) Carbohydrates are the body's primary fuel source for most functions. Our muscles, brain, and central nervous system all depend on carbohydrates for energy.

2) Carbohydrates are found in fruits, vegetables, beans, dairy products, and foods made from grain products. Sweeteners such as sugar, honey, molasses, and corn syrup also contain carbohydrates.

3) The body converts digestible (non-fiber) carbohydrates into glucose, which our cells use as fuel. Some carbohydrates, those usually referred to as simple carbohydrates, break down quickly into glucose. While others, which are usually referred to as complex carbohydrates, are slowly broken down and enter the bloodstream more gradually.

4) All carbohydrates are broken down to glucose in order to be absorbed into the bloodstream. Once in the bloodstream, insulin helps the glucose enter the body's cells. Some glucose is stored as glycogen in the liver and muscles for future use. Excess glucose is stored as fat.

THE THREE TYPES OF CARBOHYDRATES

1) *Simple carbohydrates* are composed of 1-2 sugar units that are broken down very quickly. These carbohydrates are said to cause an extreme rise in blood sugar, which then increases the release of insulin. This rise can elevate appetite and fat storage.

2) *Complex carbohydrates* or starches are made up of a chain of sugar units and are found naturally or in an unrefined state. Since they are larger units, they are broken down or digested more slowly. The unrefined carbohydrates contain more vitamins, minerals and fiber, which all promote good health. Complex carbohydrates have been shown to cause a moderate rise in blood sugar since they enter the bloodstream more gradually than simple carbohydrates. Insulin is released more steadily, which helps to stabilize appetite.

3) *Indigestible carbohydrates* are also referred to as fiber. The body is unable to digest or break down fiber into glucose, and therefore indigestible fiber is not absorbed. Since fiber is not absorbed, it is not an energy source and therefore contains no calories. However, fiber does have many health benefits.

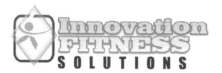

CLASSIFYING THE CARBOHYDRATES

- Fruits which contain the fruit sugar, fructose, contain primarily simple carbohydrate but also important vitamins, minerals, fiber and water. The fructose coupled with the fiber in fruit is responsible for minimal insulin response or rise in blood sugar, making fruit a healthy choice.
- Vegetables contain varying amounts of simple and complex carbohydrates, vitamins, minerals fiber and water.
- Legumes such as beans, peas, lentils and soybeans contain complex carbohydrates, fiber, vitamins, minerals and protein.
- Milk products contain simple carbohydrates along with protein, calcium and other nutrients.
- Grain products contain complex carbohydrates, fiber, vitamins, mineral and protein. The quantity is dependent upon the type of grain used and the amount of processing. Selecting whole grains whenever possible is recommended.

Each macronutrient has its own role in maintaining and energizing the body. No one macronutrient can undertake all of the body's roles, nor is any single macronutrient responsible for weight gain. By combining proteins, fats, and carbohydrates at each meal and snack, you are enabling your body and your metabolism to work most efficiently.

METABOLISM

Metabolism refers to the way that your body uses energy, which is measured in calories. Calories are used to perform vital body functions like breathing, for physical activity and for the digestion and absorption of food. The faster your metabolism works the more calories you will burn and the more weight you will lose. Timing your meals correctly allows you to ensure that your metabolism is working to full capacity.

MEAL TIMING

To reach your body composition goals, you need to know the timing of your meals and the types and amounts of food you are eating. In order for your body to use nutrients efficiently for energy, appetite control, tissue growth and repair, nutrients must be available to the body at the proper times, in the proper amounts and in the proper proportions of carbohydrate, protein and fat. Think of your metabolism like a furnace, the more often you add fuel (food) to the fire, the better it will burn. Therefore, it is better to eat every three to four hours, in order to increase the body's production of heat, caused by digestion and absorption of food, which will increase the metabolism. If you only eat 3 meals or less per day, you are depriving your body of the fuel it regularly needs to maintain your metabolism. .

Skipping breakfast can also negatively affect your energy levels. If you miss your morning meal, your energy levels will fluctuate, which will then create the tendency to overeat later in the day. In order to achieve and maintain weight loss, insulin levels must be stabilized throughout the day. Eating smaller, more frequent meals helps to achieve this stabilization and control hunger.

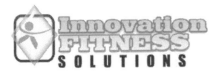

<u>**KEY POINTS:**</u>
- ✓ Eat a balanced breakfast when you wake up.
- ✓ Do not go more than 3 to 4 hours without eating (unless you are sleeping).
- ✓ Try to eat 3 meals and 2-3 snacks per day.
- ✓ Eat a snack composed of carbohydrates, protein, and fat within 45 minutes after completing a workout to help repair damaged muscle and replenish muscle glycogen (energy) stores.

Do not save the majority of your calories for one meal – your body cannot handle more than 50% of its calories at one time, and your body will end up storing the food as fat.

<u>**WATCHING YOUR PORTIONS**</u>
To accurately record the amounts of foods you are eating, it is important to know portion sizes. Many food portions nowadays are a lot larger than standard portions. For instance, a 4-inch bagel is about 4 carbohydrate servings. The NY-style bagels are twice that amount, and may contain upwards of 500 calories! To choose sensible portions, measure portions of your favorite foods once or twice, using measuring cups and spoons. You will then be aware of how much you are eating, and how it compares to a standard portion. When food scales or measuring cups are not available, you can estimate your portion sizes.

Convenient Foods for Fat Loss & Health

Splenda Flavor Blends or Splenda with Fiber
For those of us who do not drink enough water there is a tasty new way to get more in. Splenda has expanded its brand to include products for baking, as well as their new *Flavor Blends* line. There is Hazelnut, Mocha, Caramel and French Vanilla for coffee flavoring plus Orange, Lemon and Berry for water flavorings. For the caffeine addicted, we can save hundreds of calories a month by using these instead of lattes and cappuccinos.

SnackAway's Snack Foods or Weight Watchers
This falls under the category of a *"Better Bad Food Choice"*. We all succumb to temptation periodically. However, a Devil
Dog fueled bender can cost us a few hundred calories. This will not aid your weight loss endeavors. SnackAway offers all of your favorite treats in lower calorie choices that taste similar to the originals. You can get Twinkie flavor, chocolate cupcake, lemon cake and more. Weight Watchers makes a similar line of products but the cost is usually more than double.

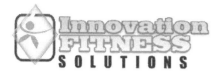
Jell-O Chocolate Pudding Snacks or Redi Whip Chocolate Whipped Crème.

Here's a recipe for low calorie, chocolate pudding that will satisfy your sweet tooth and your nutritional needs:

1.) 1 packet Fat Free/ Sugar Free Chocolate Pudding
2) 1/2 cups *Chocolate Protein Powder*
3.) 2 cups Skim Milk/ Water Combo

Baked Chips

Every manufacturer has a line of low fat or baked chips. I prefer the baked chips as some of the low fat have added fat replacements or other unnecessary additives. The chips come in all of the normal flavors. Try the cheddar and sour cream and while you are at, it buy me a bag.

Whole Wheat/ Low Calorie Pita's

These whole grain pita's and tortilla's are very low calorie (60-75 grams) and very high fiber (7-9 grams). What a great replacement for white bread.

Natural/Organic Peanut Butter

In this style peanut butter, there is none of the sugar or hydrogenated oils that are found in the regular peanut butters. If you like eating peanuts you will LOVE natural peanut butter. The annoying part is the oil separations that occurs but think of it as a workout. Grab a big knife and stir away.

Fiber 1 Bars

These things are amazingly great tasting bars. They are a bit high in sugar but some things are just worth it! They have 9 grams of fiber in only 140 calories. They come in many flavors including Peanut Butter and my favorite…chocolate chip.

High Fiber Crackers

All Bran Multi Grain Crackers come in multiple flavors and are 120-140 calories for 12 crackers (6 grams of fiber). Kashi Foods make great cereals, frozen dinners and crackers. All are great choices but this is about crackers. The Kashi crackers are 120 calories for 4 (large) with 3 grams of fiber. These are great for snacking. Lastly, there is the old stand-by...Tricuits! One of my favorite snacks is to toast Triscuits with Low Fat String Cheese and Tomato Sauce. It is like having miniature Triscuit pizzas.

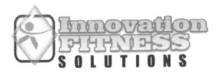

Fortified Pasta

Barilla PLUS is a great choice. Ronzoni also makes a great line of Healthy Harvest and Smart Taste Pasta. All of these have more fiber and some even have healthy additives like ALA Omega 3 fats (healthy fat). Many of the "health" brands have whole wheat options or flour blends which helps maintain that   original pasta look for those who will not eat whole wheat pasta.

Pre Measured Oatmeal

This is truly a no brainer! There are dozens of companies that make the ready to eat options. You should keep a few in your desk for breakfast in a pinch. Buy the flavored variety so you eat it! The plain is obviously healthier (less sugar) but it will not help if you will not consume it.

In the last few years, most major food brands are catching on to the health market and now you do not need to visit a specialty foods store to find these hidden gems.

Healthy Weight Loss Foods List

This list should give you a pretty good idea of the many different healthy foods you can choose from when creating your weight loss diet or just any healthy diet in general. As I mentioned before, make sure you still end up consuming the right total number of calories you figured out you should eat each day.

Good Sources of Protein

Chicken (without skin)	Swordfish	Pinto beans
Turkey (without skin)	Trout	Miso
Lean cuts of beef	Crab	Soybeans
Lean cuts of pork	Clams	Peanuts
Lean cuts of lamb	Scallops	Almonds
Lean cuts of veal	Milk (2% or skim)	Cashews
Eggs	Cottage cheese (low fat/non fat)	Hazelnuts
Egg whites	Yogurt (low fat/non fat)	Pecans
Tuna fish	Tofu	Pistachio nuts
Salmon	Black beans	Natural peanut butter
Shrimp	Garbanzo beans (aka chick peas)	Pumpkin seeds
Lobster	Kidney beans	Sunflower seeds
Flounder	Lentils	Protein powder, protein shakes
Sardines	Lima beans	and protein bars
Snapper	Navy beans	

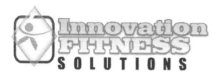

Good Sources of Carbohydrates
Brown Rice
100% whole wheat bread
100% whole wheat bagels
100% whole wheat pita bread
Whole wheat/whole grain pasta

Sweet potatoes
Yams
Oatmeal
Buckwheat
Bulgur
Bran cereals
Garbanzo beans (aka chick peas)

Kidney beans
Black beans
Lentils
Navy beans
Pinto beans
Lima Beans

(Fruits and Vegetables)
Apple
Orange
Plum
Banana
Grapes
Strawberries
Peaches
Pears
Cantaloupe

Pineapple
Broccoli
Brussels sprouts
Cabbage
Asparagus
Spinach
Lettuce
Romaine lettuce
Avocado

Cucumber
Eggplant
Tomato
Cauliflower
Celery
Bok choy
Mushrooms
Peppers
Green peas

Good Sources of Fat
Salmon
Mackerel
Herring
Anchovies
Sardines
Scallops

Halibut
Fish oil supplements
Peanuts
Almonds
Walnuts
Cashews

Natural peanut butter
Olive oil (extra-virgin)
Flax seeds
Flax seed oil
Pumpkin seeds
Sunflower seeds

The National Weight Control Registry (NWCR) is the largest ongoing study on long-term weight loss. To be included in the study, you must have lost at least 30 pounds and kept the weight off for at least one year. On average, the 5,000 participants have lost 60 pounds and maintained the weight loss for nearly six years. The range of weight loss is 30 to 300 pounds, which means any weight loss goal is possible. Interestingly, the odds appear stacked against these individuals as nearly half were overweight or obese as kids and three-quarters have at least one obese parent. So, if you think you're doomed because of your genetics, here is clear evidence to the contrary. You are NOT destined to be overweight for life and you CAN overcome it by changing certain behaviors. Here are the habits successful losers adopted to drop those unwanted pounds:

- Eat breakfast daily
- Exercise approximately 60 minutes a day
- Check weight at least once a week
- Watch less than 10 hours of television per week
- Maintain a consistent diet on weekends and weekdays
- Track food intake

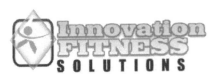

Grocery Shopping List

Here's What to Include on Your Healthy Grocery List

- Fresh vegetables and fruits should make up the largest part of your healthy foods grocery list. Vegetables and fruits have vitamins, minerals, antioxidants and they are usually low in calories. Choose a variety of fruits and vegetables that everyone in your family will enjoy.
- Most of your grain and cereal products should be made from whole grains, not from refined flours. This part of your list includes whole grain breads, whole grain pastas, and whole grain breakfast cereals. Whole grains are important for vitamins, minerals, and for fiber, which is often lacking in our diets. Read labels to look for 100% whole-grain or 100% whole-wheat to be sure you are getting whole grain products.
- Your protein and meat choices should consist mostly of fish, poultry and lean meats. Eggs, nuts, seeds and legumes are also good protein choices. Choose fresh and frozen unbreaded meats and fish. Avoid breaded, deep-fried convenience foods that you put in the oven. They are high in fats and sodium.
- Beverages should be kept simple. Water, low-fat milk, juices and herbal teas are all good choices. If you opt for soft drinks, choose diet sodas and soft drinks to avoid extra sugar.
- Dairy products should include low-fat milk, yogurt and cheese. If you do not want cows' milk, choose soy and rice beverages, calcium-fortified orange juice, or goats' milks and cheese.
- Be careful with dressings, cooking oils and condiments. They are sneaky sources of refined sugar and poor quality oils. Read labels to choose dressings made with olive oil, canola oil or walnut oil. Choose low-fat mayonnaise for your sandwiches and choose canola oil and olive oil for cooking.
- Frozen foods are a convenient way to keep vegetables on hand. There are also prepared meals that you can pop into the microwave or oven. These can be convenient and healthy if you choose low fat versions with good portion sizes. Read labels and chose frozen foods wisely. Avoid frozen pizzas, pocket-sandwiches, deep-fried appetizers, and breaded foods.
- Foods in cans and jars are also very convenient. Look for low-sodium soups, vegetables and sauces. Avoid high-fat gravies and high-calorie foods like canned spaghetti and ravioli products.
- For sandwiches, choose peanut butter or other nut butters, low-fat turkey slices or sliced roast beef. Avoid processed lunch meats, sausages and hot dogs.

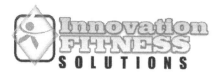

Claim	FDA Label Meanings - Requirements that must be met before using the claim in food labeling
Fat-Free	Less than 0.5 grams of fat per serving with no added fat or oil
Low fat	3 grams or less of fat per serving
Less fat	25% or less fat than the comparison food
Saturated Fat Free	Less than 0.5 grams of saturated fat and 0.5 grams of trans-fatty acids per serving
Cholesterol-Free	Less than 2 mg cholesterol per serving and 2 grams or less of saturated fat per serving
Low Cholesterol	20 mg or less cholesterol per serving and 2 grams or less of saturated fat per serving
Reduced Calorie	At least 25% fewer calories per serving than the comparison food

Examine your diet and eating patterns.

Without changing your normal eating habits, take some time to write down everything you eat today, what time you ate and then rate your energy levels after each meal from 1-5 (1 being very energetic and 5 being not energetic at all). At the end of the day, answer the following questions :

- How many times did you eat today?
- How long did you go between your meals/snacks?
- How would you rate your overall energy for the day?
- When were you the most alert and energetic?
- How do you think what you ate affected your energy levels?

Read through your answers and ask yourself if what/when you are eating is helping you or hurting you. Would you feel better if you ate smaller meals more often or do larger meals with small snacks keep you going?

Sometimes the way we eat is simply a habit that's become ingrained so ask yourself - is there a better way?

Starting Measurements:

Your first step is to record the following measurements: weight, resting heart rate, body fat and circumference measurements. Write down your numbers and be sure to write down the date. You'll use thi same chart every four weeks or so to record new numbers to track your progress.

You may also wish to get starting strength measurements as an additional way to gauge your success.

**Print out at www.InnovationFitnessSolutions.com

Right now, think of a Reason to make your heart SMILE.

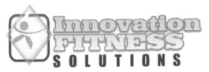

Weigh and Measure for Results

Use this chart to track your progress monthly.

Day 1	
Age	
Gender	
Height (Feet)	
Height (Inches)	
Weight (Pounds)	
Chest (Inches)	
Waist (inches)	
Body Fat	
Target Body Fat	
BMI	0.00
Target BMI	

Day 31	
Age	
Gender	
Height (Feet)	
Height (Inches)	
Weight (Pounds)	
Chest (Inches)	
Waist (inches)	
Body Fat	
Target Body Fat	
BMI	0.00
Target BMI	

Weight Loss to date:

Gender	
Height (Feet)	
Height (Inches)	
Weight (Pounds)	
Chest (Inches)	
Waist (inches)	
Body Fat	
Target Body Fat	
BMI	0.00
Target BMI	

Weight Loss to date:

Day 90	
Age	
Gender	
Height (Feet)	
Height (Inches)	
Weight (Pounds)	
Chest (Inches)	
Waist (inches)	
Body Fat	
Target Body Fat	
BMI	0.00
Target BMI	

Total Weight Loss:

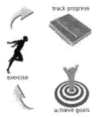
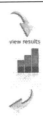

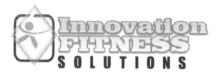
Weekly Workout Planner

Program start date	

Warm-up

Exercises	Reps	Wts (Lb)	Weeks	Frequency	Start

Strength

Exercises	Reps	Wts	Weeks	Frequency	Start

Cardio

Exercises	Reps	Wts	Weeks	Frequency	Start

Cool-down

Exercises	Reps	Wts	Weeks	Frequency	Start

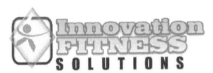

Days 1 – 30 Daily Fitness Tips

1. Get real and be specific. Write down three or four realistic goals that you can stick to. Avoid fantasy land goals that will only frustrate you.

2. Throw away all the junk, the processed, and the bingeable foods now and replace them with fresh, whole foods like lots of water and veggies.

3. Get Prepared. Buy a new pair of walking shoes and find some clothes in your closet you feel comfortable to walk in. During a lifestyle change, if you fail to plan, then you plan to fail'

4. Get support. Whether it's your best friend, spouse, or pet, it helps to have some nonjudgmental and nurturing support when trying to lose weight, especially during trying times.

5. Research has shown that keeping track of your daily exercise and food intake in a journal or notebook will increase the likelihood of success. The key is to hold you accountable.

6. Create a food free reward system. How about a new workout outfit, pair of jeans, shoes or what the heck, even a spa treatment, shopping spree, or weekend getaway? You deserve this kind of treatment when you reach your goals.

7. Make sure you have a healthy dinner consisting of lean protein, veggies, and fruit.

8. Buy a pedometer. A pedometer keeps track of how many steps you take daily. Wear it every day, around home, work, and while exercising. Your goal is to increase your steps to 10,000 or more daily!

9. Having a salad or cup of soup for starters can be a habit that pays off in pounds lost. They can curb your hunger, prevent over eating, and help you stay in control of portions.

10. Don't skip breakfast. Research shows that the most successful losers never skip it. Try to keep it balanced with some protein, a healthy carbohydrate, and a small amount of fat.

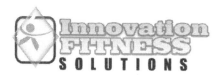

11. Have a mid afternoon snack. This will curb your appetite and provide fuel for your after work walk or workout at the gym. Figure out when your "Afternoon slump" occurs and train yourself to eat 30-45 minutes before it happens.

12. Write down your reasons for wanting to lose weight. Having clearly identified reasons helps your feeling of commitment.

13. Limit salt, caffeine, and alcohol.

14. Writing down what you eat and drink and any thoughts linked to that eating helps you become more aware of your eating habits and problem areas. Recognizing what is going on and understanding more about yourself is a powerful way to start planning changes to your diet and puts you in control.

15. Much of the eating we do when we aren't hungry, or the cravings we have, is a habit like response to a variety of triggers. These can be external, such as the sight or smell of food, or internal and emotion led, such as a response to stress, anger, boredom or emptiness. Be aware of why you are eating.

16. Setting a goal ideally includes a plan for how to achieve it, and how to overcome things that might get in the way. Writing your goals and action plans helps enormously.

17. Try to make conscious choices about what you eat, especially when tempted to overeat. For example, ask yourself, I can eat this if I want to, but do I really feel like it? You can then choose to eat it, or not, as you will have considered the consequences. Not only will it help you feel in control and achieve your goals, it will stop you feeling deprived.

18. Like a wave, cravings rise then ebb away. By waiting fifteen minutes and surfing the craving, you should find they pass away. *Drink a glass of water while waiting.*

19. You know that feeling when you really overdo the chocolate or a night out and think you've blown it so may as well give up, and keep on eating. The blow out isn't a problem, but your reaction could be. Rather than feel you have failed and give up, look at what you can learn from a bad day or week and plan to do things differently in the future. Then forgive, talk positively to yourself about what you have achieved already, and get back on track.

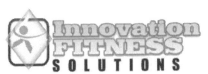

20. Eat slowly, and wait ten to fifteen minutes before taking second helpings.

21. Take in fewer calories than you expend. Few people understand this basic, simple concept. Avoid buffets.

22. Plan ahead to ensure the right foods are available at the right time. Think about breakfast, lunch, healthy snacks and an evening meal. Have some ready meals in the fridge for those emergency moments. Planning can take extra time and effort, but it will soon become a habit that will really make a difference.

23. Make meals automatically healthy, balanced and satisfying. Half fill your plate with plenty of vegetables and divide the other half between lean protein rich foods and healthy carbohydrates.

24. Eat without distractions. Don't let your best efforts to control how much you eat sabotaged by doing something else during meals.

25. We are often pressured to eat when we aren't hungry. If you really don't want to eat something, learn to say NO THANK YOU.

26. It's fine to build some favorite foods into your healthy plan. Successful people do it as it helps them avoid feeling deprived. Make sure you choose quality foods that you really feel like eating.

27. Have at least six to eight glasses or cups of water or low calorie drinks over the day. Drinking plenty helps you feel fuller and stops you confusing thirst with hunger, and eating when you really just need a drink.

28. How you think, affects how you feel, and in turn the actions you take. Believe in yourself every day. Focus on what you want, being fitter, healthier, rather than how unfit you are. Setting realistic goals and having positive expectations will make all the difference.

29. Food is everywhere and it can trigger cravings. At home, keep weakness foods out of sight, or out of the house!

30. Being able to distinguish the difference between emotional eating and physical hunger is very important. Emotional eating can cause you to overeat and subsequently gain weight. Be aware of the triggers and be ready to make positive behavior choices.

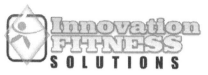

Days 31-60 Daily Fitness Tips:

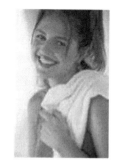

1. "Physical fitness is not only one of the most important keys to a healthy body; it is the basis of dynamic and creative intellectual activity." John F. Kennedy

2. Good flexibility in the joints can help prevent injuries through all stages of life. If you want to improve your flexibility, try activities that lengthen the muscles such as swimming or basic stretching.

3. To improve your muscle endurance, try cardio respiratory activities such as walking, jogging, bicycling, or dancing.

4. The key to making your muscles stronger is working them against resistance, whether that is from weights or gravity. If you want to gain more muscle strength, try exercises such as lifting weights or rapidly taking the stairs.

5. Ultimately, I am what I choose to be; my self-esteem follows the same path." – Anonymous

6. Whoever said physical activity is all work and no play? Participate in physical activities you enjoy!

7. Did you play any sport in High School or College? Join a sporting team with your friends, get fit and burn calories!

8. People who exercise regularly enjoy improved sleep quality. They fall asleep more quickly, sleep more deeply, awaken less often, and sleep longer.

9. Surround yourself with people and things that remind you to live a healthy lifestyle.

10. Do pushups, sit-ups or other exercises during commercial breaks. Stretch during the show!

11. Strength training is important for cardiac health because the risk of heart disease is lower when the body is leaner.

12. Enroll in a class, such as ballroom dancing or yoga or martial arts.

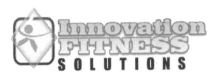

13. Want to stay young? Scientific research has shown that exercise can slow the physiological aging clock.

14. Identify what you want to accomplish with your health, strength, and weight. Set goals to plan for success.

15. At times, you will not feel like exercising. If you're just feeling a little tired or low on energy, go ahead and try to complete your routine. The workout will likely boost your energy level and your mood.

16. Stay Motivated! Surround yourself with fitness reminders at home, work, and on the computer.

17. Hang a Food Pyramid chart on your wall to remind you to eat healthily.

18. Be physically active, at a moderate intensity for at least 30 minutes most days of the week.

19. Did you overeat this weekend? Don't feel guilty about it, because it is O.K. to let go every now and then. But, recommit today to eat well and keep exercising.

20. Lift weights. It is a myth that women who lift weights will get bulky muscles.

21. Eat your fruits and vegetables." Healthy diets rich in fruits and vegetables may reduce the risk of cancer and other chronic diseases.

22. Remember to do Squats! They strengthen all of the major muscles of the lower body.

23. Calorie balance is like a scale. To remain in balance and maintain your body weight, the calories consumed (from foods) must be balanced by the calories used (in normal body functions, daily activities, and physical activity).

24. Aim for a healthy weight. People who need to lose weight should do so gradually, at a rate of one-half to two pounds per week.

25. Be active. The safest and most effective way to lose weight is to reduce calories and increase physical activity.

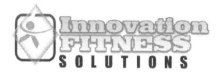

26. Regular physical activity reduces the risk for many diseases, helps control weight, and strengthens muscles, bones, and joints.

27. I am a work in progress. Focus on progress, not perfection.

28. Make sure you Journal today.

29. Park a good distance from your destination and use the opportunity to take a walk and take the stairs instead of the elevator. Small steps ultimately lead to bigger rewards.

30. Believe in yourself today!

Days 61 – 90   Daily Fitness Tips:

1. Building muscle strength and endurance through exercise will increase your total body strength and help you to maintain good posture

2. 'Next time you find yourself getting worn out during a workout think of some guy who treated you mad and made you mad - studies show that getting angry can help you work out up to thirty percent longer than usual - plus it is a healthy way to release aggressive feelings

3. Stair climbers are excellent machines for cardiovascular conditioning. They are not meant for strength training and contrary to rumors will not give you big muscles or make your butt big.

4. To get the best workout in your spinning class and avoid injury make sure the bike is adjusted right for you. Get to the class early enough to set it up and ask the instructor for help if you have problems with it.

5. Start your day with breakfast! Breakfast fills your empty tank to get you going after a long night without food. And it can help you do better in school. Easy to prepare breakfasts include cold cereal with fruit and low fat milk or whole wheat toast with peanut butter or yogurt with fruit or whole grain waffles or even last night's pizza.

ENERGY

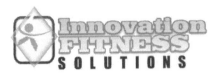

6. Listen to your body. If you find that you are dragging eat the right healthy foods that will give your body the energy that it needs.

7. Try to envision how great you will look and feel once you get in shape. Try to find a picture of someone that has the same body type and pin it up where you can look at it every day to help you see the same results you too can reach with hard work and time.

8. When you have completed your exercise regimen instead of scarfing down carbs grab some fresh fruit and water. The reason is that for a minimum of an hour after exercise the body is still breaking down fat. You need to allow the body to finish doing its job.

9. When trying to get into shape it is important to have family and friends in support. This means they need to respect your goals and not offer you wrong foods or try to pull you away from your exercise program. Explain to them how important this is to you and that you need their encouragement.

10. When you stretch your body in preparation for exercise as well as after exercise you need to stretch your mind as well. You might be wondering how and why. When your mind is relaxed your body follows. To achieve a relaxed mind listen to soothing music and relax your breathing and use visualization techniques such as imagining the most peaceful place you can think of.

11. This exercise for the backs of your legs can be done in front of the television! Sit up straight with your legs and feet and knees hip width apart. Keeping the weight evenly distributed between both feet lift your heels off the floor. Place your palms on your thighs with your elbows bent and push down as though you are trying to push your heels back onto the floor. Resist this movement with your legs. Once you have mastered this lean forward and upwards slightly to add weight.

12. That Low Fat label is not a license to eat all you want. Many low fat products are loaded with extra sugar to make up for the missing fat. This means they can be just as high in calories as their full fat counterparts. Keep portion sizes in perspective even when there is no fat involved.

13. Give yourself the gift of a healthy lifestyle by choosing wholesome foods and exercising your body on a regular basis

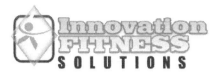

14. Want to burn major calories? Try running in the deep end of a pool wearing a flotation belt or ring for an intense water exercise workout. Use your ordinary upright running style. Deep water running is great and quite safe for athletic training and fat burning as you can work hard without the high impact that can lead to injuries.

15. Weekend workouts are not enough! Do not just save all your exercise plans for the weekend. Regular exercise throughout the week will build up your muscles slowly as well as your endurance. Vigorous exercise done only occasionally can lead to torn or strained tissue and will not do much to improve your looks or sports performance either.

16. Turn your household chores into a fitness challenge. Sweep or mop using as much energy as possible and exaggerate your arm movements. Fold your clothes and do a couple sets of squats at the same time. You might as well get fit while you make your parents happy. Just be sure the blinds are closed to prevent embarrassing moments!

17. Lunges are awesome lower body workouts. Beginners to these lower body exercises should do them without weights. Once you get stronger lunges can be done while holding dumbbells in your hands to add resistance. Start by standing with your feet together. Take a long step forward with one foot. Come down with your heel first. Then bend your front leg and sink down so the knee on your back leg is a few inches off the floor. Do not let the knee on your forward leg go past your toes or drift to either

18. A low fat diet combined with thirty minutes of aerobic exercise every other day is the best way to lose fat and get into great shape.

19. Step up to the plate and work your thighs and butt! Step ups are good leg strengthening lower body exercises you can do at home or at the gym. Find a sturdy step or bench or box that is just lower than your knee so when you put your foot on it your thigh will be parallel to the ground. If it is higher it will be hard on your knee. Too much lower and it will not be effective. Have a support you can hold on to with one hand to steady yourself during your lower body workouts. Step up with your right

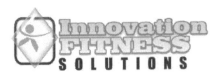

20. Here is a good lower body exercise for the hip abductor which is the muscle on the outside of your hip that moves your leg out to the side. It is one of the best exercises to tone lower body muscles. Stand on a stair step sideways with one foot on the step. Without bending the supporting leg, lower the unsupported leg a couple of inches by tilting your pelvis and then bring it back up. Repeat ten times and switch to the other leg.

21. Pay attention to how the running shoe fits. Some athletic running shoes have staggered eyelets. If your feet are narrow then use only the eyelets farthest from the tongue. For wide feet use the ones nearest the tongue.

22. Want to beat your best running time? Drink up. Running performance decreases by five to ten percent if you are dehydrated. If you have ignored all the running tips that encourage you to drink water before or during a race start listening and drinking. This is the easiest way you can find to improve your finishing time.

23. Go ahead. Buy that fuchsia running outfit! Bright colors are associated with excitement and stimulation. While you are running convince yourself to improve concentration and pick up your pace a bit when you see a red or yellow or orange object. It can be a fire hydrant or store sign or another runner's shirt.

24. To boost your metabolism and burn more calories consider alternating between two different kinds of exercise rather than just sticking to one. Trying running one day and stair climbing or swimming on another.

25. Exercise is great but you have to watch what you eat to in order to get the best results from your workouts. Working out in the gym in order to lose fat while paying no attention to what you eat is like trying to save money while charging up your credit card.

26. Being active is the enemy of unwanted weight. If you are not active and not doing anything you may just reach out for food to kill boredom. Want to get fit faster? Then keep moving and be active. Just walking up the stairs when you have the chance instead of taking the escalator can make a difference. By constantly moving you are burning fat and keeping your metabolism revved.

27. Walking is awesome exercise. Anyplace you can walk uninterrupted and build up a brisk pace is good. In the mall walking for exercise is more fun when you are window shopping!

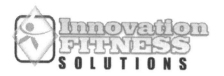
28. Wishing to lose weight? Eat your food more slowly. During a meal our brain takes about twenty minutes to signal that we are full. So if you eat too fast you might stuff in a lot of food before your brain can signal to you that your stomach is full.

29. Fitness does not have to be expensive. Ultimately any money you spend on a serious fitness routine will come back to you tenfold in health and fitness benefits and happiness. But if you are on a tight budget there should be no problem. All you need is a rope to jump or a flight of stairs to climb. And let us not forget the endless natural terrain that Mother Nature provides for us to run and hike and rollerblade on.

30. Feeling blue? That is when fitness is especially important. When you are down in the dumps grab your dancing shoes and shake your butt for health and fitness. Aerobic exercise is a proven treatment for mild depression. Or take up extreme sports if your mood is low. You will be too busy worrying about climbing down that rock wall to be depressed.

Check in with yourself.
Take at least five minutes today to flip through your journal. Read through all of it and write down the hardest challenge you've experienced so far and the easiest. Keep this information handy for the future

Reward yourself.
Take at least five minutes today and think or write about what you've accomplished so far in the Transformation Challenge. Then make a list of five things you could do to reward yourself for your hard work. Choose one thing from that list and either do it today or make plans for doing it in the future.

Fun

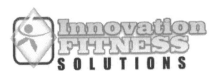

90 quick weight loss tips

1. I am a work in progress.

2. I want to be around to see my grandchildren, so I can forgo a cookie now.

3. I'll ride the wave. My cravings will disappear after 10 minutes if I turn my attention elsewhere.

4. It's more stressful to continue being fat than to stop overeating." I Eat Healthy, but I'm Overweight - What Mistakes Could I Be Making without Realizing It?

5. The best portion of high-calorie foods is the smallest one. The best portion of vegetables is the largest one. Period.

6. A bag of frozen vegetables heated in the microwave, topped with 2 tablespoons of Parmesan cheese and 2 tablespoons of chopped nuts

7. A healthy frozen entree with a salad and a glass of 1 percent milk

8. A peanut butter sandwich on whole wheat bread with a glass of 1 percent milk and an apple

9. A smoothie made with fat-free milk, frozen fruit, and Protein Powder

10. Add just one fruit or veggie serving daily. Get comfortable with that, and then add an extra serving until you reach 8 to 10 a day.

11. Are you the kind of person who does better if you make up your mind to do without sweets and just not have those around? Or are you going to do better if you have a limited amount of sweets every day? KNOW what will work for you long term.

12. As obvious as it sounds, don't stand near the food at parties. Make the effort, and you'll find you eat less.

13. At a buffet? Eating a little of everything guarantees high calories. Decide on three or four things, only one of which is high in calories. Save that for last so there's less chance of overeating.

14. Brush your teeth right after dinner to remind you: No more food.

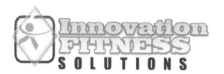

15. Cereal, fruit, and fat-free milk makes a good meal anytime.

16. Change your nighttime schedule. It will take effort, but it will pay off. You need something that will occupy your mind and hands.

17. Cut back on or cut out caloric drinks such as soda, sweet tea, lemonade, etc. People have lost weight by making just this one change. If you have a 20-oz bottle of Coca-Cola every day, switch to Diet Coke. You should lose 20 lbs in a year.

18. Dance to music with your family in your home. One dietitian reported that when she asks her patients to do this, initially they just smile, but once they've done it, they say it is one of the easiest ways to involve the whole family in exercise.

19. How Can I Control a Raging Sweet Tooth? Dilute juice with water.

20. Doctor your veggies to make them delicious: Dribble maple syrup over carrots, and sprinkle chopped nuts on green beans.

21. Don't "graze" yourself fat. You can easily munch 600 calories of pretzels or cereal without realizing it.

22. Don't forget that vegetable soup counts as a vegetable.

23. Drink cold unsweetened raspberry tea. It tastes great and keeps your mouth busy.

24. Drinking too little can hamper your weight loss efforts. That's because dehydration can slow your metabolism by 3 percent, or about 45 fewer calories burned a day, which in a year could mean weighing 5 pounds more. The key to water isn't how much you drink; it's how frequently you drink it. Small amounts sipped often work better than 8 ounces gulped down at once.

25. Eat breakfast, lunch, and dinner. The large majority of people who struggle with night eating are those who skip meals or don't eat balanced meals during the day. This is a major setup for overeating at night.

26. Eat the low-cal items on your plate first, and then graduate. Start with salads, veggies, and broth soups, and eat meats and starches last. By the time you get to them, you'll be full enough to be content with smaller portions of the high-calorie choices.

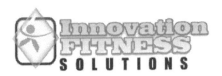

27. Eat without engaging in any other simultaneous activity. No reading, watching TV, or sitting at the computer.

28. Eat your evening meal in the kitchen or dining room, sitting down at the table.

29. Eat your sweets, just eat them smart! Carve out about 150 calories per day for your favorite sweet. That amounts to about an ounce of chocolate, half a modest slice of cake, or 1/2 cup of regular ice cream.

30. Eating late at night won't itself cause weight gain. It's how many calories -- not when you eat them -- that counts.

31. Eating out? Halve it, and bag the rest. A typical restaurant entree has 1,000 to 2,000 calories, not even counting the bread, appetizer, beverage and dessert.

32. Eating pasta like crazy: A serving of pasta is 1 cup, but some people routinely eat 4 cups.

33. Follow the Chinese saying: "Eat until you are eight-tenths full."

34. For the duration of the holidays, wear your snuggest clothes that don't allow much room for expansion. Wearing sweats is out until January.

35. Get calories from foods you chew, not beverages. Have fresh fruit instead of fruit juice.

36. Give it away! After company leaves, give away leftover food to neighbors, doormen, or delivery people or take it to work the next day.

37. Have the smallest fast-food burger (with mustard and ketchup, not mayo) and a no-cal beverage. Then at home, have an apple or baby carrots.

38. Here's another reason to keep level-headed all the time: Pennsylvania State University research has found that women less able to cope with stress -- shown by blood pressure and heart rate elevations -- ate twice as many fatty snacks as stress-resistant women did, even after the stress stopped (in this case, 25 minutes of periodic jackhammer-level noise and an unsolvable maze).

39. Eat at home.

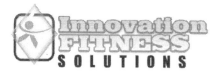

40. If you're eating at night due to emotions, you need to focus on getting in touch with what's going on and taking care of yourself in a way that really works. Find a nonfood method of coping with your stress.

41. If you're famished by 4PM and have no alternative but an office vending machine, reach for the nuts. The same goes if your only choices are what's available in the hotel minibar.

42. If your family thinks they need a very sweet treat every night, try to strike a balance between offering healthy choices and allowing them some "free will." Compromise with low-fat ice cream and fruit, or sometimes just fruit with whipped cream.

43. Instead of whole milk, switch to 1 percent. If you drink one 8-oz glass a day, you'll lose 5 lbs in a year.

44. Juice has as many calories, ounce for ounce, as soda. Set a limit of one 8-oz glass of fruit juice a day.

45. Keep lean sandwich fixings on hand: whole wheat bread, sliced turkey, reduced-fat cheese, tomatoes, and mustard with horseradish.

46. Keep seven bags of your favorite frozen vegetables on hand. Mix any combination, microwave, and top with your favorite low-fat dressing. Enjoy 3 to 4 cups a day. Makes a great quick dinner.

BMI Calculator

Exercise Tips

Weight Loss Tips

Calorie Counter

Calorie Calculator

Drinking Water

47. Limit alcohol to weekends.

48. Make exercise a nonnegotiable priority.

49. Heat up a can of good soup.

50. Make eating purposeful, not mindless. Whenever you put food in your mouth, peel it, unwrap it, plate it and sit. Engage all of the senses in the pleasure of nourishing your body.

51. Make sure your plate is half veggies and or fruit at both lunch and dinner.

52. Mix three different cans of beans and some diet Italian dressing. Eat this three-bean salad all week.

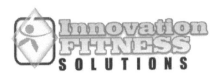

90 Days to A New You

53. Nothing's less appetizing than a crisper drawer full of mushy vegetables. Frozen vegetables store much better, plus they may have greater nutritional value than fresh. Food suppliers typically freeze veggies just a few hours after harvest, locking in the nutrients. Fresh veggies, on the other hand, often spend days in the back of a truck before they reach your supermarket.

54. Once in a while, have a lean, mean salad for lunch or dinner, and save the meal's calories for a full dessert.

55. Overeating is not the result of exercise. Vigorous exercise won't stimulate you to overeat. It's just the opposite. Exercise at any level helps curb your appetite immediately following the workout.

56. Prebagged salad topped with canned tuna, grape tomatoes, shredded reduced-fat cheese, and low-cal Italian dressing

57. Precooked chicken strips and microwaved frozen broccoli topped with Parmesan cheese

58. Precut fruit for a salad and add yogurt.

59. Put a sign on the kitchen and refrigerator doors: "Closed after Dinner."

60. Really hate veggies? Relax. If you love fruits, eat plenty of them; they are just as healthy (especially colorful ones such as oranges, mangoes and melons).

61. Rediscover the sweet potato. Sweet potato fries are really tasty.

62. Remember, eat before you meet. Have this small meal before you go to any parties: a hardboiled egg, apple and a thirst quencher (water, seltzer, diet soda, tea).

63. Resolve never to supersize your food portions -- unless you want to supersize your clothes.

64. Scramble eggs in a nonstick skillet. Pop some asparagus in the microwave, and add whole wheat toast. If your cholesterol levels are normal, you can have seven eggs a week!

65. See what you eat. Plate your food instead of eating out of the jar or bag.

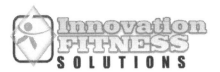

66. Sit when you eat.

67. *Sitting at a computer may help you slim down. When researchers at Brown University School of Medicine put 92 people on online weight-loss programs for a year, those who received weekly e-mail counseling shed 5 1/2 more pounds than those who got none. Counselors provided weekly feedback on diet and exercise logs, answered questions, and cheered them on. Most major online diet programs offer many of these features.*

68. Skipping breakfast will leave you tired and craving naughty foods by midmorning. To fill up healthfully and tastefully, try this sweet, fruity breakfast full of antioxidants. In a blender, process 1 c nonfat plain or vanilla yogurt, 1 1/3 c frozen strawberries (no added sugar), 1 peeled kiwi, and 1 peeled banana. Pulse until mixture is milkshake consistency. Makes one 2-cup serving; 348 calories and 1.5 fat grams.

69. Skipping meals: Many healthy eaters "diet by day and binge by night."

70. Snacking on bowls of nuts. Nuts are healthy but dense with calories. Put those bowls away, and use nuts as a garnish instead of a snack.

71. Spend the extra few dollars to buy vegetables that are already washed and cut up.

72. Eat breakfast. It helps you eat fewer total calories throughout the day. Take your lunch to work.

73. Think yoga's too serene to burn calories? Think again. You can burn 250 to 350 calories during an hour-long class (that's as much as you'd burn from an hour of walking)! Plus, you'll improve muscle strength, flexibility, and endurance.

74. Try a veggie sandwich from Subway.

75. Try two weeks without sweets. It's amazing how your cravings vanish

76. Try these smart little sweets: sugar-free hot cocoa, frozen red grapes, fudgsicles, sugar-free gum, Nutri-Grain chocolate fudge twists, Tootsie Rolls, and hard candy.

77. Use prebagged baby spinach everywhere: as "lettuce" in sandwiches, heated in soups, wilted in hot pasta, and added to salads.

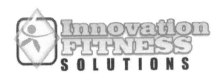

78. Tune in to an audio book while you walk. It'll keep you going longer and looking forward to the next walk -- and the next chapter!

79. Use a salad plate instead of a dinner plate.

80. Use mustard instead of mayo. Try Spicy Mustard for variety.

81. Walk around the mall three times before you start shopping.

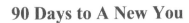

82. When dining out, make it automatic: Order one dessert to share.

83. According to researchers at Cornell University. In a recent study, they discovered that people not only underestimate the number of calories in wholesome fare, but they also consume substantially larger portions of it.

84. *Avoid the Vending Machines.* If you remember to prepare in advance and bring healthy snacks, this should not be an issue. If, however, you forgot, remember to look for calorically cheaper, more filling items. If there is a dried fruit and nut mix opt for that, or try soy chips if they are available.

85. If your body is deficient in any nutrient, the body will break down muscle tissue to release more nutrients. As a result, your metabolism may slow down slightly due to a reduction in muscle mass. Take your Multi-Vitamin.

86. Control your portions and prevent overeating by using smaller plates and bowls. Weight loss is about portion control. Make your meals seem larger by putting away your dinner plates and only using your salad plates. Also, try pouring your drinks into taller/thinner glasses. Studies show that this has a similar effect for liquids.

87. Negative thinking leads to negative results and a loss of motivation. Tell yourself everyday: "Just for today I will focus on the positives."

88. Track your progress. Maintain a record of your starting statistics and all throughout your journey. Refer to these during low times to boost your motivation back to where it should be. We all fall sometimes. Winners get up.

89. Have Nutrition Bars available for snacks so you do not miss meals and overeat.

90. Believe in yourself today.

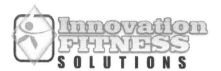

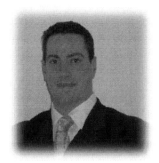

About the Author:

Robert J. DeVito is the President and Founder of **Innovation Fitness Solutions**.
IFS coaches thousands of clients annually through live coaching and phone/internet coaching.

Robert has been serving the fitness industry in various capacities (Personal Trainer, Weight Management Specialist, National Certification Educator, consultant and entrepreneur) for more than fifteen years. He has had the honor of certifying more than 7500 Fitness Professionals and working with 200+ health clubs. Robert has presented at Conferences for Club Industry (CIE), the National Fitness Business Alliance (NFBA) and the New England Health, Racquet and Sports Association (NEHRSA) on topics ranging from business to personal training and weight management.

Robert has made a significant impact in the health, wellness and fitness industry through his unique approach to *solution based programming* for health club members and an innovative approach to complete health and fitness. His passionate commitment to education has made him a highly sought after presenter, consultant and author.
He has taught health club staff members, management and owners how to completely integrate all departments of their business to be more profitable, productive and member-centric.

His mission is simple: to Innovate the way fitness is presented, sold and serviced.

**For a complete resume and biography please visit

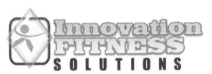

Help for those who want individual attention:

What is Weight Loss Coaching?

Weight Loss Coaching helps you to achieve results and keep the weight off for good, giving you a body that looks and feels fantastic. You probably know what you need to do to lose weight and be healthier; yet doing it is often the hard part. For instance, you know that you should only eat when you're hungry or drink plenty of water each day. Working with a coach helps you to find a way to do these things and to keep with them permanently.

Your Weight Loss Success Coach supports you and encourages you to take the steps towards losing weight and being healthier. We are your partners and offer you the opportunity to look at your weight loss and health from different perspectives. When you have someone who really believes in you, you will succeed faster.

What can you expect from coaching?
+ We will listen to you
+ Challenge you
+ Want the best for you
+ Keep you focused and on track

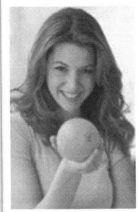

Results Driven Programs with Care
+ Discover solutions to your weight loss problems
+ We keep the emphasis on habits and solutions not foods or calories.
+ We will focus on taking great care of you.
+ Working with you to make a plan to accomplish what you want.
+ Faster, more efficient results.
+ Long Term Weight Loss.
+ No more confusion and yo-yo weight loss.

Features:
+ 12 Week Program. (Flexible Structure)
+ 30 minute Phone/Internet Coaching
+ Weekly Educational Articles
+ Daily Motivational/Inspirational Quotes and Updates
+ On-Line Menu Planning, Journaling
+ Exercise Programming
+ (Surprise Exercise/ Out of Gym Activity)
+ Individual Programming and Coaching
+ Realistic, Progressive and Maintainable Programs
+ Call 201-951-8080 to schedule your Complimentary Session

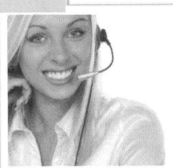

Made in the USA
Charleston, SC
04 January 2010